Clinical Hematology Atlas

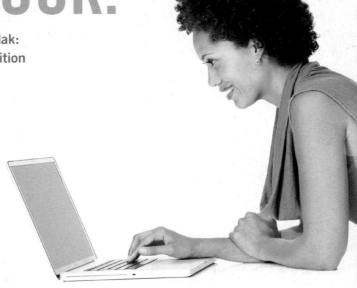

Fifth Edition

Clinical Hematology Atlas

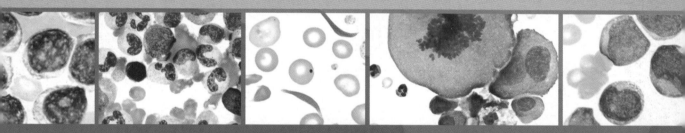

Bernadette F. Rodak, MS, MT(ASCP)SH
Professor Emeritus
Clinical Laboratory Science Program
Department of Pathology and Laboratory Medicine
Indiana University School of Medicine
Indianapolis, Indiana

Jacqueline H. Carr, MS, MT(ASCP)SH
Former Laboratory Manager
Department of Pathology and Laboratory Medicine
Indiana University Health
Indianapolis, Indiana

ELSEVIER

ELSEVIER

3251 Riverport Lane
St. Louis, Missouri 63043

CLINICAL HEMATOLOGY ATLAS, FIFTH EDITION   ISBN: 978-0-323-32249-2

Notices

Knowledge and best practice in this field are constantly changing. As new research and experience broaden our understanding, changes in research methods, professional practices, or medical treatment may become necessary.

Practitioners and researchers must always rely on their own experience and knowledge in evaluating and using any information, methods, compounds, or experiments described herein. In using such information or methods they should be mindful of their own safety and the safety of others, including parties for whom they have a professional responsibility.

With respect to any drug or pharmaceutical products identified, readers are advised to check the most current information provided (i) on procedures featured or (ii) by the manufacturer of each product to be administered, to verify the recommended dose or formula, the method and duration of administration, and contraindications. It is the responsibility of practitioners, relying on their own experience and knowledge of their patients, to make diagnoses, to determine dosages and the best treatment for each individual patient, and to take all appropriate safety precautions.

To the fullest extent of the law, neither the Publisher nor the authors, contributors, or editors, assume any liability for any injury and/or damage to persons or property as a matter of products liability, negligence or otherwise, or from any use or operation of any methods, products, instructions, or ideas contained in the material herein.

Previous editions copyrighted 2013, 2009, 2004, and 1999.

International Standard Book Number: 978-0-323-32249-2

Library of Congress Cataloging-in-Publication Data
Rodak, Bernadette F., author.
   Clinical hematology atlas / Bernadette F. Rodak, Jacqueline H. Carr.
     —Fifth edition.
       p. ; cm.
   Includes index.
   ISBN 978-0-323-32249-2 (pbk. : alk. paper)
   I. Carr, Jacqueline H., author. II. Title.
   [DNLM: 1. Hematologic Diseases–diagnosis–Atlases. 2. Hematologic Diseases–pathology–Atlases. WH 17]
   RB145
   616.1'5–dc23
                                                                      2015036694

Executive Content Strategist: Kellie White
Content Development Manager: Laurie Gower
Content Development Specialist: Karen Turner
Publishing Services Manager: Julie Eddy
Project Manager: Abigail Bradberry
Design Direction: Julia Dummitt

Printed in Canada
Last digit is the print number: 11 10   9   8   7

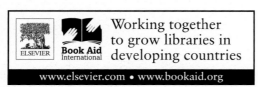

To our husbands,
Robert Hartman
and
Charles Carr,
daughters,
Kimberly Carr Mayrose
and
Alexis Carr,
*and all of our colleagues who have encouraged us
to continue to publish this atlas in its concise format*

REVIEWERS

Steven Marionneaux, MS, MT(ASCP)
Manager, Clinical Hematology Laboratories
Memorial Sloan Kettering Cancer Center
New York, New York
Adjuct Assistance Professor, Clinical Laboratory Sciences
Rutgers, The State University of New Jersey
Newark, New Jersey

Alisa J. Petree, MHSM, MLS(ASCP)cm
Professor/Clinical Coordinator
McLennan Community College
Waco, Texas

B ecause the emphasis of an atlas is morphology, the *Clinical Hematology Atlas* is intended to be used with a textbook, such as *Rodak's Hematology*, fifth edition, that addresses physiology and diagnosis along with morphology. This atlas is designed for a diverse audience that includes clinical laboratory science students, medical students, residents, and practitioners. It is also a valuable resource for clinical laboratory practitioners who are being retrained or cross-trained in hematology. It is not intended to be a detailed, comprehensive manual for diagnosis.

In this concise format, every photomicrograph and word has been evaluated for value to the microscopist. All superfluous information has been excluded in an attempt to maintain focus on significant microscopic findings while correlating this information with clinical diagnosis. What started as a primer for Clinical Laboratory Science students with no previous hematology education has evolved into an internationally recognized reference for multiple levels of expertise, from entry level to practicing professionals.

ORGANIZATION

As is frequently expounded, morphology on a peripheral blood film is only as good as the quality of the smear and the stain. Chapter 1 reviews smear preparation, staining, and the appropriate area in which to evaluate cell distribution and morphology. A table that summarizes the morphology of leukocytes found in a normal differential, along with multiple examples of each cell type, facilitates early instruction in blood smear review.

Chapter 2 schematically presents hematopoietic features of cell maturation. General cell maturation, along with an electron micrograph with labeled organelles, will help readers correlate the substructures with the appearance of cells under light microscopy. Visualizing normal cellular maturation is essential to the understanding of disease processes. This correlation of schematic, electron micrograph, and Wright-stained morphology is carried throughout the maturation chapters. Figure 2-1 has been formatted to reflect recent hematopoietic theory. In addition, the chart aids readers in recognizing the anatomical sites at which each stage of maturation normally occurs.

Chapters 3 to 9 present the maturation of each cell line individually, repeating the respective segment of the overall hematopoietic scheme from Chapter 2, to assist the student in seeing the relationship of each cell line to the whole. In these chapters, each maturation stage is presented as a color print, a schematic, and an electron micrograph. A description of each cell, including overall size, nuclear-to-cytoplasmic ratio, morphologic features, and reference ranges in peripheral blood and bone marrow, serves as a convenient summary. The final figure in each of these chapters summarizes lineage maturation by repeating the hematopoietic segment with the corresponding photomicrographs. Multiple nomenclatures for erythrocyte maturation are used to accommodate use in multiple settings and demographic groups.

Chapters 10 to 12 present discrete cellular abnormalities of erythrocytes, that is, variations in size, color, shape, and distribution, as well as inclusions found in erythrocytes. Each variation is presented along with a description of the abnormality, or composition of the inclusion, and associated disorders.

Because diseases are often combinations of the cellular alterations, Chapter 13 integrates morphologic findings into the diagnostic features of disorders primarily affecting erythrocytes.

In Chapter 14, nuclear and cytoplasmic changes in leukocytes are displayed and correlated with non-malignant leukocyte disorders.

Diseases of excessive or altered production of cells may be caused by maturation arrest, asynchronous development, or proliferation of one cell line, as presented in Chapters 15 to 19. Cytochemical stains are presented with disorders in which they are useful.

The therapeutic use of myeloid growth factors causes morphologic changes that mimic severe infections or malignancies. Chapter 20 presents examples of peripheral blood morphology following G-CSF or GM-CSF. It is the authors' design that the cellular defects in leukocyte disorders be visually compared with the process of normal hematopoiesis for a more thorough comprehension of normal and altered development. Readers are encouraged to refer to the normal hematopoiesis illustration, Figure 2-1, for comparison of normal and abnormal cells and the progression of diseases.

Microorganisms, including parasites, may be seen on peripheral blood smears. A brief photographic overview is given in Chapter 21. Readers are encouraged to consult a microbiology reference, such as Mahon CM, Lehman DC, Manuselis G: *Textbook of Diagnostic Microbiology*, fifth edition, for a more detailed presentation.

Chapter 22 includes photomicrographs that are not categorized into any one particular area, such as fat cells, mitotic figures, metastatic tumor cells, and artifacts.

Chapter 23 describes findings expected in the peripheral blood of neonates, including anticipated variations in morphology and cellular distribution. Comparison of the hematogone, normal for newborns, with the blast cell of acute leukemia is included.

Chapter 24 is intended to be an overview of the most frequent microscopic findings in body fluids. It is not proposed as a comprehensive review of the cytology of human body fluids, but rather a quick reference for the beginning microscopist as well as the seasoned professional.

As with the third edition and fourth editions, the fifth edition features spiral binding, making the atlas more convenient when used at the microscope bench.

All of these chapters combine into what we believe is a comprehensive and valuable resource for any clinical laboratory. The quality of the schematic illustrations, electron micrographs, and color photographs stand for themselves. We hope that this atlas will enrich the learning process for the student and serve as an important reference tool for the practitioner.

EVOLVE

The Evolve website provides free materials for both students and instructors. Instructors have access to an electronic image collection featuring all of the images from the atlas. Students and instructors have access to summary tables, student review exercises, and additional photos for identification.

Bernadette F. Rodak
Jacqueline H. Carr

ACKNOWLEDGMENTS

From inception to completion we have had a great deal of assistance and encouragement from the faculty and staff of the Department of Pathology and Laboratory Medicine, Indiana University School of Medicine. The following individuals have "gone the extra mile" to help us continue to realize our dream: **George Girgis**, MT(ASCP), for sharing his incredible collection of body fluid slides and his expertise in both blood cell and body fluid morphology; **Linda Marler** and **Jean Siders** for their technical assistance with digital photography and digital editing; and **Linda Marler** and **Carla Clem**, faculty members in the Clinical Laboratory Science program, for their support and patience during this endeavor. Carla also provided authoritative comments on images and helped us determine which images were classic examples. A particular thank you goes out to our families for their understanding during the many hours that we spent away from them while pursuing this goal.

A special thank you goes to the professionals at Elsevier who navigated us through the production of this atlas. We would especially like to thank **Laurie Gower,** Content Development Manager, **Karen Turner,** Content Development Specialist, **Rebecca Corradetti,** Developmental Editor at Spring Hollow Press, **Abigail Bradberry,** Project Manager, and **Julie Eddy**, Publishing Services Manager.

CONTENTS

CHAPTER 1

INTRODUCTION TO PERIPHERAL BLOOD FILM EXAMINATION

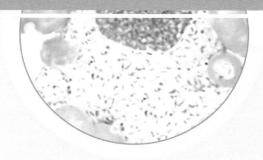

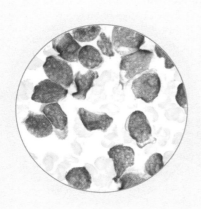

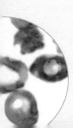

A properly prepared blood film is essential to accurate assessment of cellular morphology. A variety of methods are available for preparing and staining blood films, the most common of which are discussed in this atlas. It is beyond the scope of this atlas to discuss other methodologies; however, detailed descriptions of these procedures can be found in textbooks on hematology, such as Keohane, Smith, and Walenga's *Rodak's Hematology: Clinical Principles and Applications*.

WEDGE FILM PREPARATION

MAKING THE PERIPHERAL BLOOD FILM

Although some automated analyzers prepare and stain blood films according to established criteria, manual blood film preparation is still used in many places. The wedge film is a convenient and commonly used technique for making peripheral blood films. This technique requires at least two 3 × 1-inch (75 × 25-mm) clean glass slides. High-quality, beveled-edge microscope slides are recommended. One slide serves as the blood film slide, and the other as the spreader slide. These can then be reversed to prepare a second film. A drop of ethylenediaminetetraacetic acid (EDTA) anticoagulated blood about 3 mm in diameter is placed at one end of the slide. Alternatively, a similar size drop of blood directly from a finger or heel puncture is acceptable. The size of the drop of blood is important. Too large a drop creates a long or thick film, and too small a drop often makes a short or thin film. In preparing the film, the technician holds the pusher slide securely in front of the drop of blood at a 30- to 45-degree angle to the film slide (Figure 1-1, *A*). The pusher slide is pulled back into the drop of blood and held in that position until the blood spreads across the width of the slide (Figure 1-1, *B*). It is then quickly and smoothly pushed forward to the end of the film slide, creating a wedge film (Figure 1-1, *C*). It is important that the whole drop of blood is picked up and spread. Moving the pusher slide forward too slowly accentuates poor leukocyte distribution by pushing larger cells, such as monocytes and granulocytes, to the very ends and sides of the film. Maintaining a consistent angle between the slides and an even, gentle pressure is essential. It is frequently necessary to adjust the angle between the slides to produce a satisfactory film. For higher than normal hematocrit, the angle between the slides must be lowered so that the film is not too short and thick. For extremely low hematocrit, the angle must be raised. A well-made peripheral blood film (Figure 1-2) has the following characteristics:

1. About two-thirds to three-fourths of the length of the slide is covered by the film.
2. It is slightly rounded at the feather edge (thin portion), not bullet shaped.
3. Lateral edges of the film should be visible. The use of slides with chamfered (beveled) corners may facilitate this appearance.
4. It is smooth without irregularities, holes, or streaks.
5. When the slide is held up to light, the feather edge of the film should have a "rainbow" appearance.
6. The whole drop is picked up and spread.

Figure 1-3 shows examples of unacceptable films.

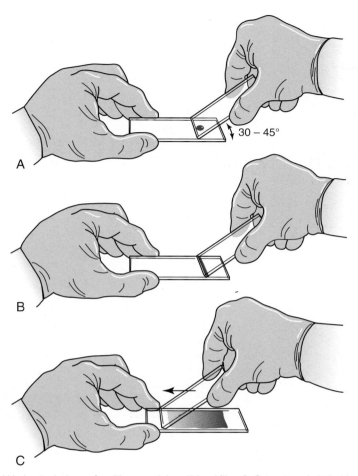

FIGURE 1–1 Wedge technique of making a peripheral blood film. **A**, Correct angle to hold spreader slide. **B**, Blood spread across width of slide. **C**, Completed wedge film.
(From Keohane E.A., Smith L., Walenga J. (Eds.) (2016). *Rodak's hematology: clinical principles and applications*. (5th ed.). St. Louis: Saunders Elsevier.)

FIGURE 1–2 Well-made peripheral blood film.
(From Keohane E.A., Smith L., Walenga J. (Eds.) (2016). *Rodak's hematology: clinical principles and applications*. (5th ed.). St. Louis: Saunders Elsevier.)

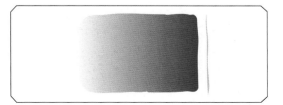

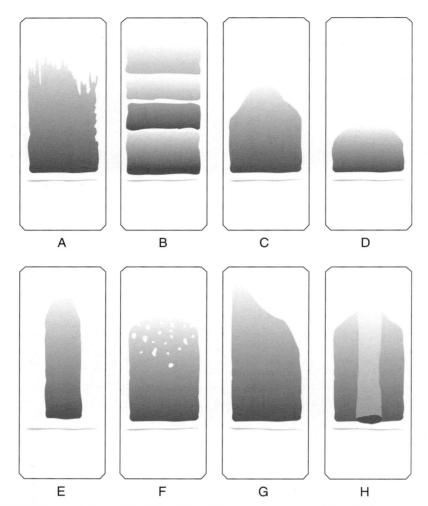

FIGURE 1–3 Unacceptable peripheral blood films. Slide appearances associated with the most common errors are shown, but note that a combination of causes may be responsible for unacceptable films. **A**, Chipped or rough edge on spreader slide. **B**, Hesitation in forward motion of spreader slide. **C**, Spreader slide pushed too quickly. **D**, Drop of blood too small. **E**, Drop of blood not allowed to spread across the width of the slide. **F**, Dirt or grease on the slide; may also be caused by elevated lipids in the blood specimen. **G**, Uneven pressure on the spreader slide. **H**, Time delay; drop of blood began to dry. (From Keohane E.A., Smith L., Walenga J. (Eds.) (2016). *Rodak's hematology: clinical principles and applications*. (5th ed.). St. Louis: Saunders Elsevier.)

STAINING OF PERIPHERAL BLOOD FILMS

The purpose of staining blood films is to identify cells and recognize morphology easily through the microscope. Wright or Wright–Giemsa stains are the most commonly used for peripheral blood and bone marrow films. These stains contain both eosin and methylene blue and are therefore termed *polychrome stains*. The colors vary slightly from laboratory to laboratory, depending on the method of staining.

Slides must be allowed to dry thoroughly before staining. The cells are fixed to the glass slide by the methanol in the stain. Staining reactions are pH dependent, and the actual staining of the cellular components occurs when a buffer (pH 6.4) is added to the stain. Free methylene blue is basic and stains acidic cellular components, such as RNA, blue. Free eosin is acidic and stains basic components, such as hemoglobin or eosinophilic granules, red. Neutrophils have cytoplasmic granules that have a neutral pH and accept some characteristics from both stains. Details for specific methods of staining peripheral blood and bone marrow films, including automated methods, may be found in a standard textbook of hematology.

An optimally stained film (Figure 1-4) has the following characteristics:

1. The red blood cells (RBCs) should be pink to salmon.
2. Nuclei are dark blue to purple.
3. Cytoplasmic granules of neutrophils are lavender to lilac.
4. Cytoplasmic granules of basophils are dark blue to black.
5. Cytoplasmic granules of eosinophils are red to orange.
6. The area between the cells should be colorless, clean, and free of precipitated stain.

A well-stained slide is necessary for accurate interpretation of cellular morphology. The best staining results are obtained from freshly made slides that have been prepared within 2 to 3 hours of blood collection. Box 1-1 lists common reasons for poorly stained slides and may be used as a guide when troubleshooting.

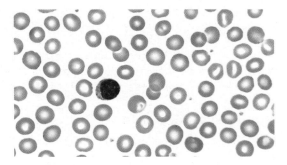

FIGURE 1–4 Optimally stained peripheral blood film demonstrating the appropriate area in which to perform the white blood cell differential and morphology assessment and the platelet estimate. Only the center of the field is shown; an entire field would contain 200 to 250 red blood cells (original ×1000).

BOX 1-1

Troubleshooting Poorly Stained Blood Films

First Scenario

Problems
- Red blood cells appear gray
- White blood cells are too dark
- Eosinophil granules are gray, not orange

Causes
- Stain or buffer too alkaline (most common)
- Inadequate rinsing
- Prolonged staining
- Heparinized blood sample

Second Scenario

Problems
- Red blood cells too pale or red color
- White blood cells barely visible

Causes
- Stain or buffer too acidic (most common)
- Underbuffering (time too short)
- Over-rinsing

From Keohane E.A., Smith L., Walenga J. (Eds.) (2016). *Rodak's hematology: clinical principles and applications.* (5th ed.). St. Louis: Saunders Elsevier.

PERIPHERAL FILM EXAMINATION

10× EXAMINATION

Examination of the blood film is a multistep process. Begin the film examination with a scan of the slide using the $10\times$ or low-power objective (total magnification $= 100\times$). This step is necessary to assess the overall quality of the film, including abnormal distribution of RBCs, suggesting the presence of rouleaux or autoagglutination, and/or the presence of a disproportionate number of large nucleated cells such as monocytes or neutrophils at the edges of the film. If the latter exists, another film should be prepared. In addition, the $10\times$ film examination allows for the rapid detection of large abnormal cells such as blasts, reactive lymphocytes, and parasites.

40× OR 50× EXAMINATION

Using the $40\times$ (high dry) objective or the $50\times$ oil objective ($400\times$ and $500\times$ total magnification, respectively), find an area of the film in which the RBCs are evenly distributed and barely touching one another (two or three cells may overlap; Figure 1-5). Scan eight to ten fields in this area of the film, and determine the average number of white blood cells (WBCs) per field. Although an exact factor varies with the make and model of microscope, in general, an approximate WBC count per cubic millimeter can be determined by multiplying the average number of WBCs per high-power field by 2000 (if $40\times$ is used), or 2500 (if $50\times$ is used).

FIGURE 1-5 Correct area of blood film in which to evaluate cellular distribution and perform white blood cell estimate (×400).

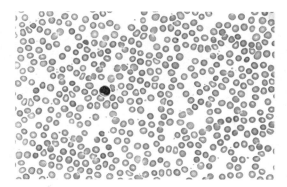

This estimate is a useful quality-control tool for validating WBC counts from hematology analyzers. Any discrepancy between the instrument WBC count and the slide estimate must be resolved. Some reasons for discrepancies include the presence of WBC or platelet clumps, fibrin strands, severe RBC agglutination, cryoprecipitate, and giant platelets, in addition to a mislabeled film, a film made from the wrong patient's sample, and an instrument malfunction.

100× EXAMINATION

The next step in film evaluation is to perform the WBC differential. This is done in the same area of the film as the WBC estimate but using the 100 × oil immersion objective (1000 × total magnification). When the correct area of the film from a patient with a normal RBC count is viewed, about 200 to 250 RBCs per oil immersion field are seen (see Figure 1-4). Characteristically, the differential count includes counting and classifying 100 consecutive WBCs and reporting these classes as percentages. The differential count is performed in a systematic manner using the "battlement" track (Figure 1-6), which minimizes WBC distribution errors. The results are reported as percentages of each type of WBC seen during the count. An example of a WBC differential count is 3% bands, 55% segmented neutrophils, 30% lymphocytes, 6% monocytes, 4% eosinophils, and 2% basophils (Table 1-1). Any WBC abnormalities, such as toxic changes, Döhle bodies, reactive lymphocytes, and Aüer rods, are also reported. When present, nucleated red blood cells (NRBCs) are counted and reported as number of NRBCs per 100 WBCs. The RBC, WBC, platelet morphology evaluation, and platelet estimates are also performed under the 100 × oil immersion objective. RBC inclusions, such as Howell-Jolly bodies, and WBC

FIGURE 1-6 "Battlement" pattern for performing a white blood cell differential. (From Keohane E.A., Smith L., Walenga J. (Eds.) (2016). *Rodak's hematology: clinical principles and applications.* (5th ed.). St. Louis: Saunders Elsevier.)

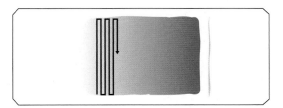

TABLE 1-1

Cells Found in a Normal White Blood Cell Differential

Cell Type	Cell Size (μm)	Nucleus	Chromatin	Cytoplasm	Granules	Adult Reference Range Peripheral Blood (%)	Cells × 10⁹/L
Segmented neutrophil (Seg), polymorphonuclear neutrophil (Poly, PMN)	10 to 15	2 to 5 lobes connected by thin filaments without visible chromatin	Coarsely clumped	Pale pink, cream colored, or colorless	1°: Rare 2°: Abundant	50 to 70	2.3 to 8.1
Band neutrophil (Band)	10 to 15	Constricted, but chromatin must be visible within the thinnest part	Coarsely clumped	Pale blue to pink	1°: Few 2°: Abundant	0 to 5	0.0 to 0.6
Lymphocyte (Lymph)	7 to 18*	Round to oval; may be slightly indented; occasional nucleoli	Condensed to deeply condensed	Scant to moderate; sky blue	± Few azurophilic	20 to 40	0.8 to 4.8
Monocyte (Mono)	12 to 20	Variable; may be round, horseshoe, or kidney shaped; often has folds producing "brainlike" convolutions	Moderately clumped; lacy	Blue-gray; may have pseudopods; vacuoles may be absent or numerous	Many fine granules, frequently giving the appearance of ground glass	3 to 11	0.5 to 1.3
Eosinophil (Eos)	12 to 17	2 to 3 lobes connected by thin filaments without visible chromatin	Coarsely clumped	Cream to pink; may have irregular borders	1°: Rare 2°: Abundant red to orange, round	0 to 5	0.0 to 0.4
Basophil (Baso)	10 to 14	Usually two lobes connected by thin filaments without visible chromatin	Coarsely clumped	Lavender to colorless	1°: Rare 2°: Lavender to dark purple; variable in number with uneven distribution; may obscure nucleus or wash out during staining, giving the appearance of empty areas in cytoplasm	0 to 1	0.0 to 0.1

*The difference in size from small to large lymphocyte is primarily a result of a larger amount of cytoplasm. See Chapter 9 for more detailed information on lymphocyte size.
1°, primary; *2°*, secondary.

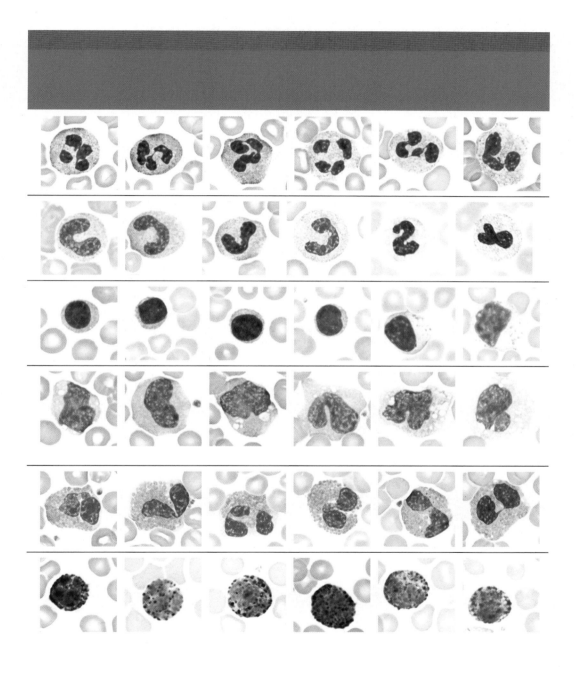

inclusions, such as Döhle bodies, can be seen at this magnification. Each laboratory should have established protocols for standardized reporting of abnormalities.

Evaluation of the RBC morphology is an important aspect of the film evaluation and is used in conjunction with the RBC indices to describe cells as normal or abnormal in size, shape, and color. Each laboratory should establish a standard reporting protocol. Most laboratories use concise statements describing overall RBC morphology that is consistent with the RBC indices. The microscopic evaluation of RBC morphology must be congruent with the information given by the automated hematology analyzer. If not, discrepancies must be resolved before reporting patient results.

The final step in the performance of the differential count is the estimation of the platelet number. This is done under the $100\times$ oil immersion objective. In an area of the film where RBCs barely touch, the number of platelets in five to ten oil immersion fields is counted. The average number of platelets is multiplied by 20,000 to provide an estimate of the total number of platelets per cubic millimeter. This estimate is reported as adequate if the estimate is consistent with a normal platelet count, decreased if below the lower limit of normal for that laboratory, and increased if above the upper limit of normal. A general reference range is 150,000 to $450,000/mm^3$ ($150–450 \times 10^9/L$). When a patient is extremely anemic or has erythrocytosis, a more involved formula for platelet estimates may be used.

The estimate can be compared with an automated platelet count as an additional quality-control measure. If the estimate and the instrument platelet count do not agree, discrepancies must be resolved. Some causes for discrepancies include the presence of giant platelets, many schistocytes (red blood cell fragments), and platelet satellitism. Notably, high-quality $40\times$ or $50\times$ oil immersion objectives can be used by the experienced technologist to perform the differential analysis of the blood film. However, all abnormal findings must be verified under the $100\times$ objective.

SUMMARY

A considerable amount of valuable information can be obtained from properly prepared, stained, and evaluated peripheral blood films. Many laboratories use films made by the wedge technique from EDTA anticoagulated blood and stained with Wright or Wright-Giemsa stain. The films should be evaluated in a systematic manner using first the $10\times$, then $40\times$ high dry or $50\times$ oil, and finally the $100\times$ oil immersion objectives on the microscope. WBC differential and morphology and the RBC morphology and platelet estimate are included in the film evaluation.

CHAPTER 2

HEMATOPOIESIS

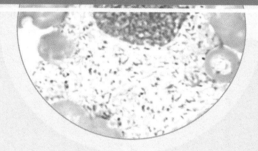

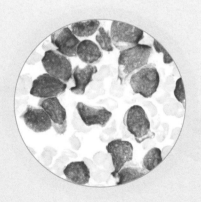

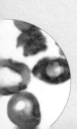

ematopoiesis is a vigorous process of blood cell production and maturation that occurs primarily in the bone marrow in the adult. The process begins with the pluripotential hematopoietic stem cell (multipotent progenitor), which is capable of proliferation, replication, and differentiation. In response to cytokines (growth factors), the pluripotential stem cell will differentiate into a common myeloid or common lymphoid progenitor. Both the myeloid and lymphoid progenitors maintain their pluripotential capacity. The lymphoid progenitor proliferates and differentiates into T, B, and natural killer cells. The myeloid progenitor proliferates and differentiates into granulocyte, monocyte, erythrocyte, and megakaryocyte lineages. To this point in maturation, none of these stem cells can be morphologically identified, although it is postulated that they appear similar to a small resting lymphocyte. The blue shaded area in Figure 2-1 highlights the stem cell populations. Each lineage and maturation stage will be presented in detail in the following chapters.

Hematopoiesis is a dynamic continuum. Cells gradually mature from one stage to the next and may be between stages when viewed through the microscope. In general, the cell is then identified as the more mature stage. General morphological changes in blood cell maturation are demonstrated in Figure 2-2.

Figures 2-3, *A* and *B*, illustrate cell ultrastructure. A review of organelles will facilitate correlation of morphological maturation with cell function. This topic is explored in depth in hematology textbooks, such as Keohane, Smith, and Walenga's Rodak's Hematology: Clinical Principles and Applications. Table 2-1 delineates the location, appearance, and function of individual organelles.

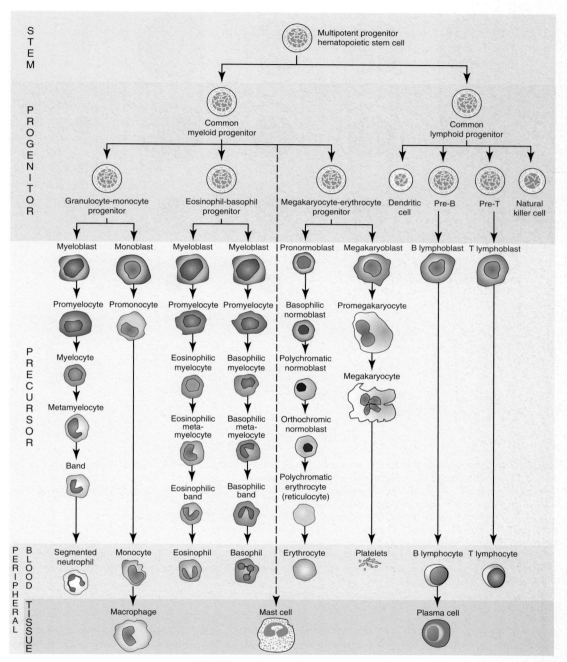

FIGURE 2–1 Chart of hematopoiesis.

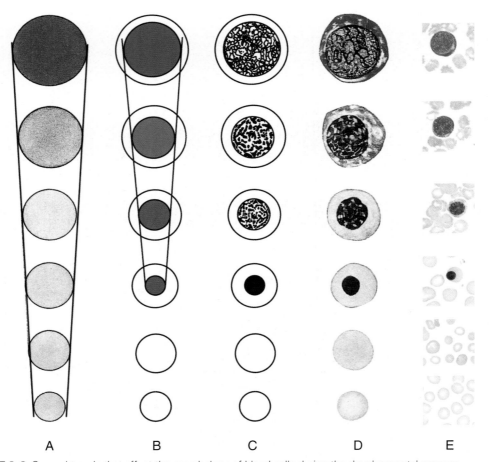

A   B   C   D   E

FIGURE 2–2 General trends that affect the morphology of blood cells during the developmental process.
A, Cell diameter decreases and cytoplasm becomes less basophilic.
- An exception to the diameter decreasing is observed in the granulocytic series, the promyelocyte may be larger than its precursor, the myeloblast (see Chapter 5).
- In the erythroid series, hemoglobin development in the cytoplasm imparts a pink/salmon color.

B, Nuclear diameter decreases (N:C ratio decreases). Nuclear color changes from purplish red to dark blue.
C, Nuclear chromatin becomes coarser, clumped, and condensed.
- Nucleoli disappear.
- In the granulocytic series, the nuclear shape changes and the nucleus becomes segmented. Granules appear in cytoplasm (see Chapter 5).
- In the erythroid series, the nucleus becomes fully condensed and is ejected.

D, Composite of changes during maturation process.
E, Representative cells from the erythroid series, demonstrating maturation changes.
(Modified from Diggs, L.W., Sturm, D., Bell, A. (1985). *The morphology of human blood cells.* (5th ed.). Abbott Park: Abbott Laboratories. Reproduction of *The Morphology of Human Blood Cells* has been granted with approval of Abbott Laboratories, all rights reserved by Abbott Laboratories.)

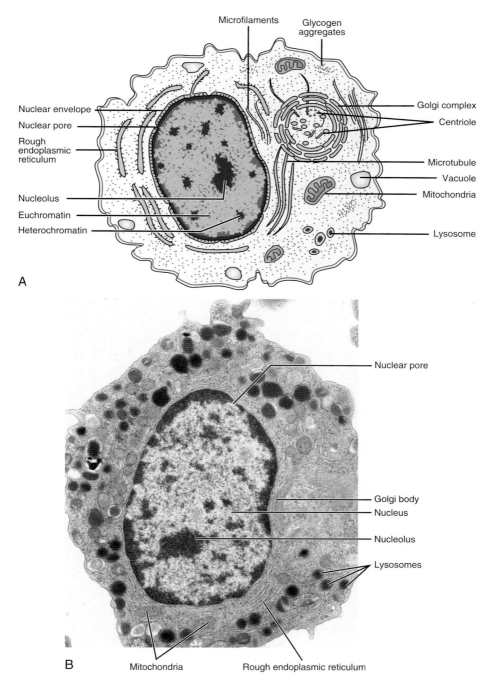

FIGURE 2–3 A, Schematic of electron micrograph. **B**, Electron micrograph with labeled organelles.
(**A**, From Keohane E.A., Smith L, Walenga J. (Eds.) (2016). *Rodak's hematology: clinical principles and applications*.
(5th ed.). St. Louis: Saunders Elsevier.)

TABLE 2-1

Summary of Cellular Components and Functions

Organelle	Location	Appearance and Size	Function	Comments
Membranes: plasma, nuclear, mitochondrial, endoplasmic reticulum	Outer boundary of cell, nucleus, endoplasmic reticulum, mitochondria, and other organelles	Usually a lipid bilayer consisting of proteins, cholesterol, phospholipids, and polysaccharides; membrane thickness varies with cell or organelle	Separates various cellular components; facilitates and restricts cellular exchange of substances	Membrane must be resilient and flexible
Nucleus	Within cell	Usually round or oval but varies depending on cell; varies in size; composed of DNA	Control center of cell containing the genetic blueprint	Governs cellular activity and transmits information for cellular control
Nucleolus	Within nucleus	Usually round or irregular in shape; 2 to 4 μm in size; composed of RNA; there may be 1 to 4 within nucleus	Site of synthesis and processing of ribosomal RNA	Appearance varies with activity of the cells; larger when cell is actively involved in protein synthesis
Golgi body	Next to nucleus	System of stacked, membrane-bound, flattened sacs; horseshoe shaped; varies in size	Involved in modifying and packaging macromolecules for secretion	Well developed in cells with large secretion responsibilities
Endoplasmic reticulum	Randomly distributed throughout cytoplasm	Membrane-lined tubules that branch and connect to nucleus and plasma membrane	Stores and transports fluids and chemicals	Two types: smooth with no ribosomes, rough with ribosomes on the surface
Ribosomes	Free in cytoplasm; outer surface of rough endoplasmic reticulum	Small granule, 100 to 300 Å; composed of protein and nucleic acid	Site of production of proteins, such as enzymes and blood proteins	Large proteins are synthesized from polyribosomes (chains of ribosomes)
Mitochondria	Randomly distributed in cytoplasm	Round or oval structures; 3 to 14 nm in length; 2 to 10 nm in width; membrane has two layers; inner layer has folds called *cristae*	Cell's "powerhouse"; make ATP, the energy source for the cell	Active cells have more present than do inactive ones
Lysosomes	Randomly distributed in cytoplasm	Membrane-bound sacs; size varies	Contain hydrolytic enzymes for cellular digestive system	If the membrane breaks, hydrolytic enzymes can destroy the cell
Microfilaments	Near nuclear envelope and component of mitotic process	Small, solid structure approximately 5 nm in diameter	Support cytoskeleton and motility	Consist of actin and myosin (contractile proteins)
Microtubules	Cytoskeleton, near nuclear envelope and component part of centriole near Golgi body	Hollow cylinder with protofilaments surrounding the outside tube; 20 to 25 nm in diameter, variable length	Maintains cell shape, motility, and mitotic process	Produced from tubulin polymerization; make up mitotic spindles and part of structure of centriole
Centriole	In centrosome near nucleus	Cylinders; 150 nm in diameter, 300 to 500 nm in length	Serves as insertion point for mitotic spindle fibers	Composed of nine sets of triplet microtubules

(From Keohane E.A., Smith L, Walenga J. (Eds.) (2016). *Rodak's hematology: clinical principles and applications.* (5th ed.). St. Louis: Saunders Elsevier.)
ATP, Adenosine triphosphate; *DNA,* deoxyribonucleic acid; *RNA,* Ribonucleic acid.

CHAPTER 3

ERYTHROCYTE MATURATION

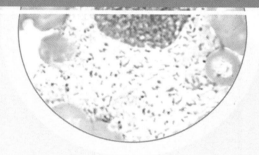

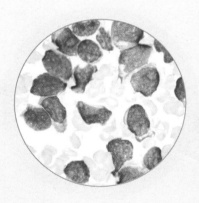

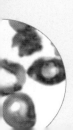

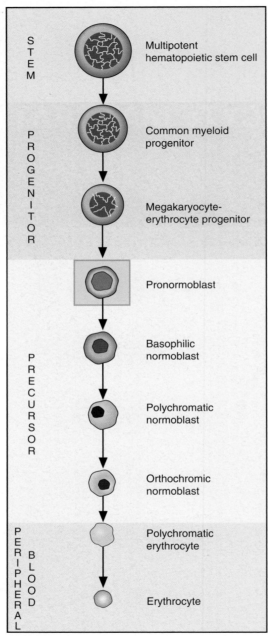

FIGURE 3–1 Erythrocyte sequence: pronormoblast.

All photomicrographs are × 1000 original magnification with Wright-Giemsa staining unless stated otherwise.

PRONORMOBLAST
Proerythroblast
Rubriblast

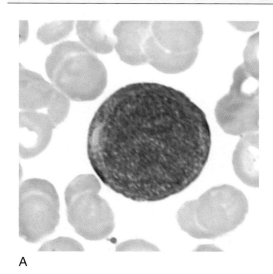

A

FIGURE 3–2A Pronormoblast.

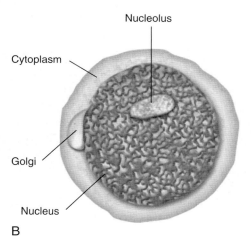

B

FIGURE 3–2B Schematic of pronormoblast.

SIZE: 12 to 20 μm

NUCLEUS: Round to slightly oval
Nucleoli: 1 to 2
Chromatin: Fine

CYTOPLASM: Dark blue; may have prominent Golgi

N:C RATIO: 8:1

REFERENCE INTERVAL:
Bone Marrow: 1%
Peripheral Blood: 0%

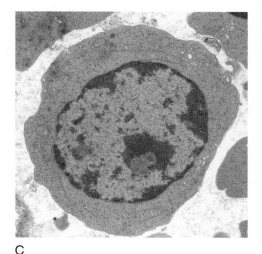

C

FIGURE 3–2C Electron micrograph of pronormoblast (×15,575).

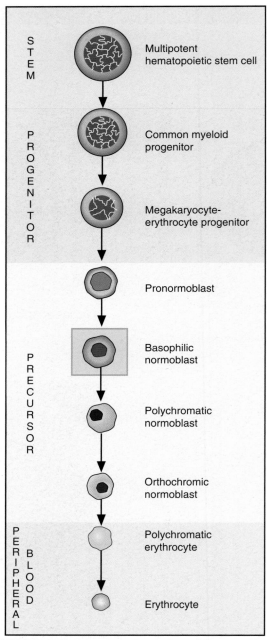

FIGURE 3–3 Erythrocyte sequence: basophilic normoblast.

BASOPHILIC NORMOBLAST
Basophilic Erythroblast
Prorubricyte

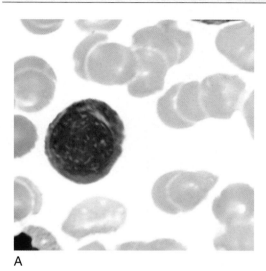

FIGURE 3–4A Basophilic normoblast.

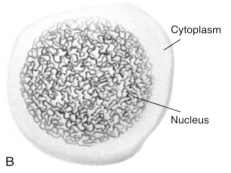

FIGURE 3–4B Schematic of basophilic normoblast.

SIZE: 10 to 15 μm

NUCLEUS: Round to slightly oval
Nucleoli: 0 to 1
Chromatin: Slightly condensed

CYTOPLASM: Dark blue

N:C RATIO: 6:1

REFERENCE INTERVAL:
Bone Marrow: 1% to 4%
Peripheral Blood: 0%

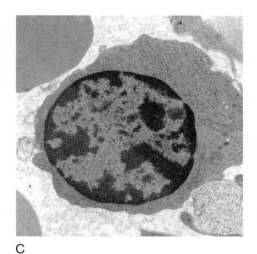

FIGURE 3–4C Electron micrograph of basophilic normoblast (×15,575).

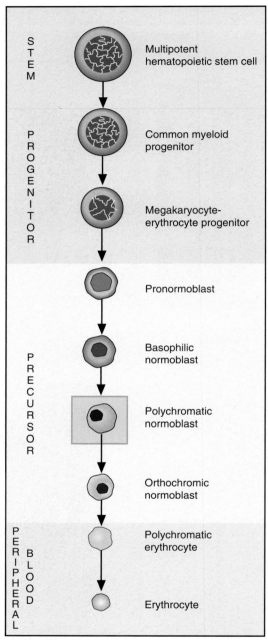

STEM

Multipotent
hematopoietic stem cell

PROGENITOR

Common myeloid
progenitor

Megakaryocyte-
erythrocyte progenitor

PRECURSOR

Pronormoblast

Basophilic
normoblast

Polychromatic
normoblast

Orthochromic
normoblast

PERIPHERAL BLOOD

Polychromatic
erythrocyte

Erythrocyte

FIGURE 3–5 Erythrocyte sequence: polychromatic normoblast.

POLYCHROMATIC NORMOBLAST
Polychromatic Erythroblast
Rubricyte

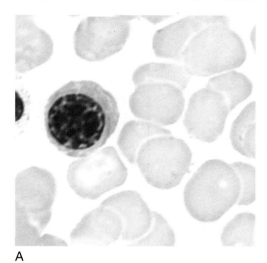

A

FIGURE 3–6A Polychromatic normoblast. The blue color of the cytoplasm is becoming gray-blue as hemoglobin is produced.

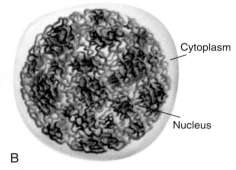

B

FIGURE 3–6B Schematic of polychromatic normoblast.

SIZE: 10 to 12 μm

NUCLEUS: Round
Nucleoli: None
Chromatin: Quite condensed

CYTOPLASM: Gray-blue as a result of hemoglobinization

N:C RATIO: 4:1

REFERENCE INTERVAL:
Bone Marrow: 10% to 20%
Peripheral Blood: 0%

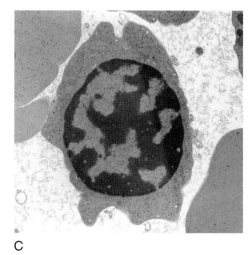

C

FIGURE 3–6C Electron micrograph of polychromatic normoblast (×15,575).

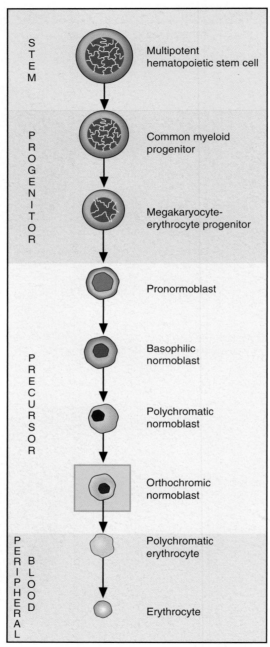

FIGURE 3–7 Erythrocyte sequence: orthochromic normoblast.

ORTHOCHROMIC NORMOBLAST
Orthochromic Erythroblast
Metarubricyte

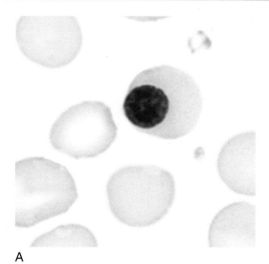

A

FIGURE 3–8A Orthochromic normoblast. The gray-blue color of the cytoplasm is becoming salmon as more hemoglobin is produced.

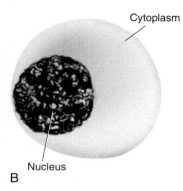

B

FIGURE 3–8B Schematic of orthochromic normoblast.

SIZE: 8 to 10 μm

NUCLEUS: Round
Nucleoli: 0
Chromatin: Fully condensed

CYTOPLASM: More pink or salmon than blue

N:C RATIO: 0.5:1

REFERENCE INTERVAL:
Bone Marrow: 5% to 10%
Peripheral Blood: 0%

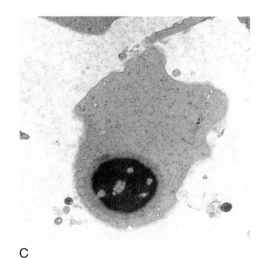

C

FIGURE 3–8C Electron micrograph of orthochromic normoblast (×20,125).

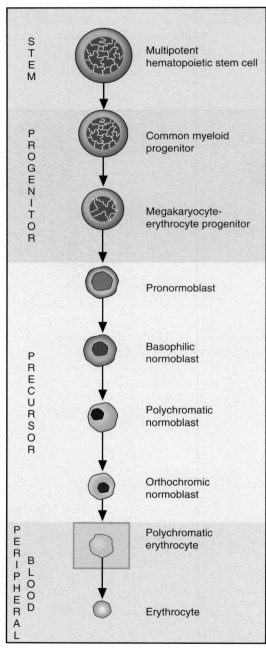

STEM

PROGENITOR

PRECURSOR

PERIPHERAL BLOOD

Multipotent hematopoietic stem cell

Common myeloid progenitor

Megakaryocyte-erythrocyte progenitor

Pronormoblast

Basophilic normoblast

Polychromatic normoblast

Orthochromic normoblast

Polychromatic erythrocyte

Erythrocyte

FIGURE 3–9 Erythrocyte sequence: polychromatic erythrocyte (reticulocyte).

POLYCHROMATIC ERYTHROCYTE
Diffusely Basophilic Erythrocyte
Reticulocyte

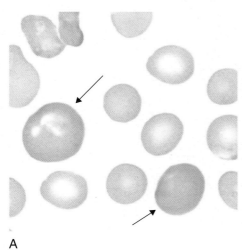

A

FIGURE 3–10A Polychromatic erythrocyte. Sometimes appears "lumpy" and larger than mature red blood cells. Slight gray-blue color persists while the cell attains full hemoglobinization.

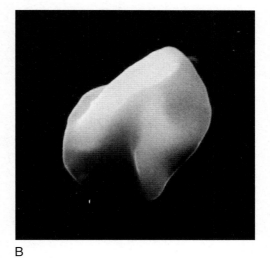

B

FIGURE 3–10B Scanning electron micrograph of polychromatic erythrocyte (×5000). Note that the reticulocyte is a very deformable cell, giving it a "lumpy" appearance by scanning electron microscopy.

SIZE: 8 to 8.5 μm

NUCLEUS: Absent
Nucleoli: NA
Chromatin: NA

CYTOPLASM: Color is slightly more blue/purple than the mature erythrocyte

N:C RATIO: NA

REFERENCE INTERVAL:
Bone Marrow: 1%
Peripheral Blood: 0.5% to 2.0%

NOTE: When stained with supravital stain (e.g., new methylene blue), polychromatic erythrocytes appear as reticulocytes (contain precipitated ribosomal material; see Figure 12–5A).

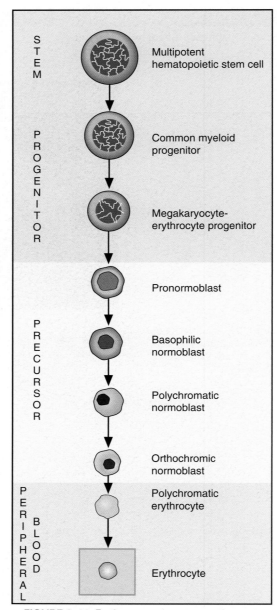

FIGURE 3–11 Erythrocyte sequence: erythrocyte.

ERYTHROCYTE

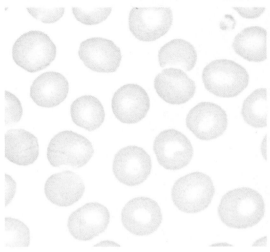

A

FIGURE 3–12A Erythrocyte. The mature erythrocyte has lost the blue-gray color and is salmon colored as hemoglobinization is complete.

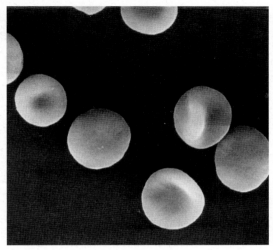

B

FIGURE 3–12B Scanning electron micrograph of erythrocyte (×2500).

SIZE: 7 to 8 μm

NUCLEUS: Absent
Nucleoli: NA
Chromatin: NA

CYTOPLASM: Salmon with central pallor of about one-third of the diameter of the cell

N:C RATIO: NA

REFERENCE INTERVAL:
Bone Marrow: NA
Peripheral Blood: Predominant cell type

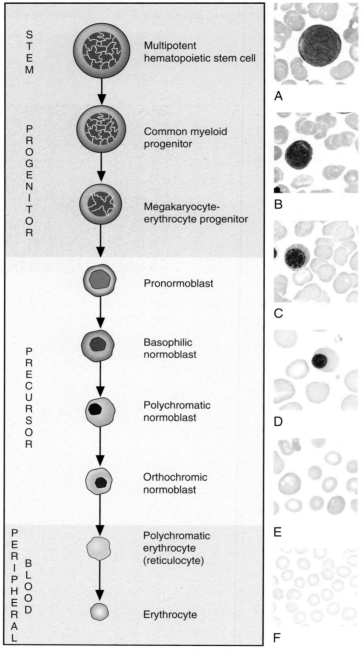

FIGURE 3–13 Erythrocyte sequence with **A**, pronormoblast; **B**, basophilic normoblast; **C**, polychromatic normoblast; **D**, orthochromic normoblast; **E**, polychromatic erythrocyte; **F**, erythrocyte.

CHAPTER 4

MEGAKARYOCYTE MATURATION

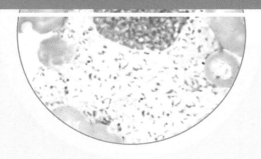

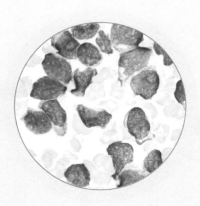

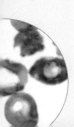

latelets arise from the megakaryocyte. Megakaryocytes are among the largest cells in the body and mature by a unique process called *endomitosis*. In endomitosis, the nucleus is duplicated but there is no cell division, resulting in a polyploid cell. Megakaryocyte nuclei may have from 2 to 32 lobes and in unusual cases may have up to 64 lobes. Megakaryocytes develop copious cytoplasm, which differentiates into platelets. Platelets have several types of granules that can be visualized by electron microscopy. The granules are highly specialized. Refer to a hematology textbook, such as *Rodak's Hematology: Clinical Principles and Applications,* for further discussion.

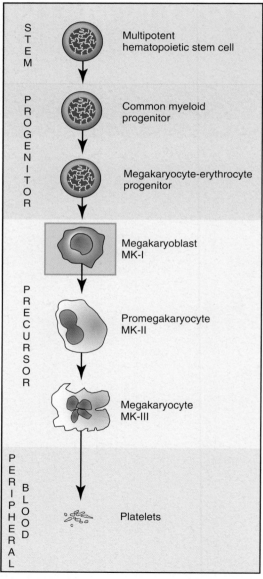

FIGURE 4–1 Megakaryocyte sequence: megakaryoblast MK-I.

MEGAKARYOBLAST (MK-I)

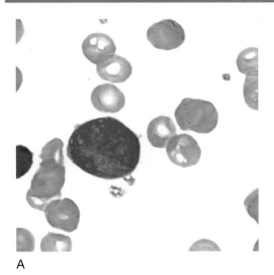

A

FIGURE 4–2A Megakaryoblast, MK-I: bone marrow (×1000).

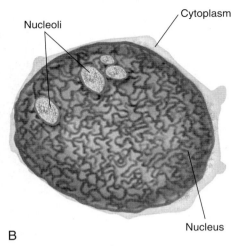

B

FIGURE 4–2B Megakaryoblast, schematic.

SIZE: 10 to 24 μm

NUCLEUS: Round
Nucleoli: 2 to 6
Chromatin: Homogeneous, loosely organized

CYTOPLASM: Basophilic
Granules: Absent by Wright stain

N:C RATIO: 3:1

REFERENCE INTERVAL:
Bone Marrow: 20% of megakaryocyte precursors in bone marrow
Peripheral Blood: 0%

NOTE: The megakaryoblast appears similar to the myeloblast and pronormoblast. Identification by morphology alone is not advisable.

All photomicrographs are × 1000 original magnification with Wright–Giemsa staining unless stated otherwise.

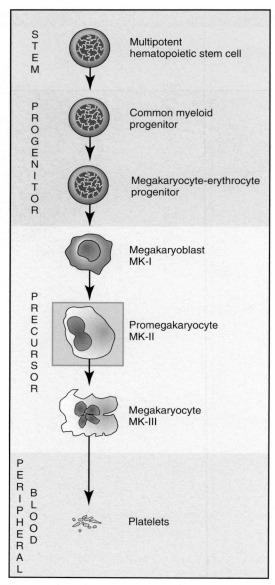

FIGURE 4–3 Megakaryocyte sequence: promegakaryocyte (MK-II).

PROMEGAKARYOCYTE (MK-II)

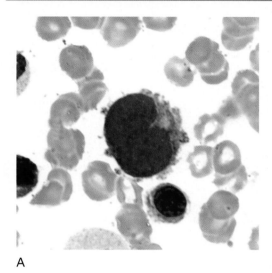

A

FIGURE 4–4A Promegakaryocyte, MK-II: bone marrow (×1000).

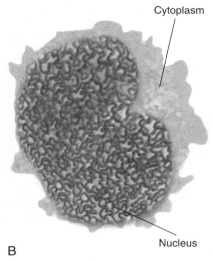

B

FIGURE 4–4B Promegakaryocyte, schematic.

SIZE: 15 to 40 µm

NUCLEUS: Indented
Nucleoli: Variable
Chromatin: Condensed

CYTOPLASM: Basophilic
Granules: Present

N:C RATIO: 1:2

REFERENCE INTERVAL:
Bone Marrow: 25% of megakaryocyte precursors in bone marrow
Peripheral Blood: 0%

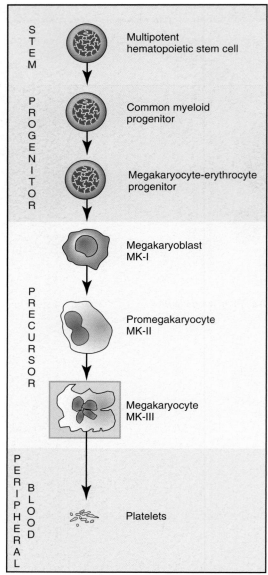

FIGURE 4–5 Megakaryocyte sequence: megakaryocyte (MK-III).

MEGAKARYOCYTE (MK-III)

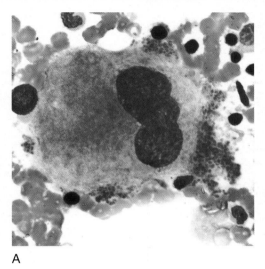

A

FIGURE 4–6A Megakaryocyte, MK III: bone marrow (×500).

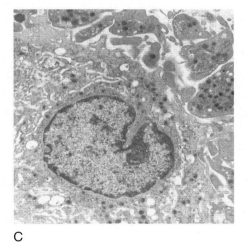

FIGURE 4–6B Megakaryocyte, MK-III, schematic.

Labels: Platelets, Nucleus, Cytoplasm, Platelets

SIZE: 20 to 90 µm

NUCLEUS: 2 to 32 lobes (8 lobes: most common)

NOTE: The size of the cell varies according to the number of lobes present.

CYTOPLASM: Blue to pink; abundant
Granules: Reddish blue; few to abundant

N:C RATIO: Variable

REFERENCE INTERVAL:
Bone Marrow: 5 to 10 per 10 × objective (× 100 magnification)
1 to 2 per 50 × objective (× 500 magnification)

NOTE: Megakaryocytes are usually reported as adequate, increased, or decreased and not as a percentage.

Peripheral Blood: 0%

C

FIGURE 4–6C Electron micrograph of megakaryocyte (×16,500).

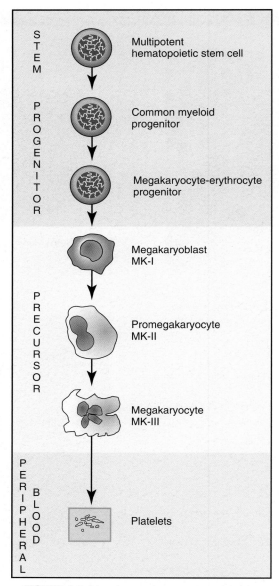

FIGURE 4–7 Megakaryocyte sequence: platelets.

PLATELET

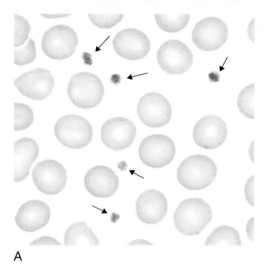

A

FIGURE 4–8A Platelet: peripheral blood (×1000).

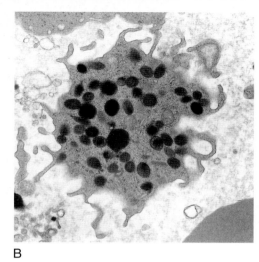

B

FIGURE 4–8B Electron micrograph of platelet (×28,750).

SIZE: 2 to 4 μm

NUCLEUS: NA

CYTOPLASM: Light blue to colorless
Granules: Red to violet, abundant

N:C RATIO: NA

REFERENCE INTERVAL:
Bone Marrow: NA
Peripheral Blood: 7 to 25 per 100× oil immersion field (×1000 magnification)

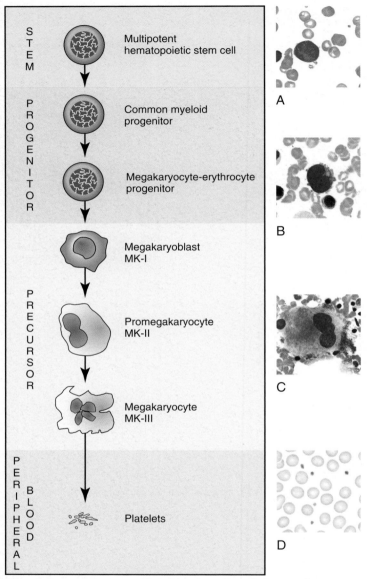

FIGURE 4–9 Megakaryocyte sequence with **A**, Megakaryoblast. **B**, Promegakaryocyte. **C**, Megakaryocyte. **D**, Platelet.

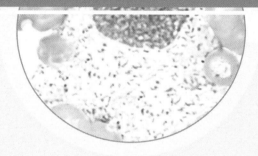

CHAPTER 5

NEUTROPHIL MATURATION

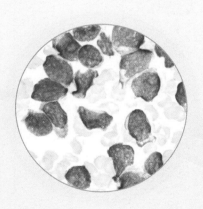

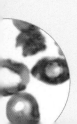

The common myeloid progenitor creates three types of progenitors: granulocytes/monocytes, eosinophils/basophils, and erythrocytes/megakaryocytes. Each of these divides and matures into cells known as *blasts*, one for each cell line. However, it is not possible to differentiate the various blasts at the light microscope level. This chapter addresses neutrophil maturation. (See Chapter 7 for discussion of eosinophils and Chapter 8 for discussion of basophils.)

As the cells mature from the myeloblast to the promyelocyte, there is a slight increase in size, in contrast with size variation in other cell lineages. At the promyelocyte stage, the chromatin in the nucleus becomes slightly coarser than the myeloblast, and primary burgundy-colored (azurophilic) granules appear in the cytoplasm. As the cell divides and matures to a myelocyte, chromatin becomes coarser and condensed, and secondary (specific) granules appear in the cytoplasm beginning at the Golgi apparatus and spreading throughout the cytoplasm. Primary granules are still present but less visible on a Wright-stained smear because of a chemical change in the membranes. It is often possible at the myelocyte stage to see the area of the Golgi apparatus, which appears as a clearing close to the nucleus. The specific secondary granules differentiate the cell into neutrophil, eosinophil, and basophil. The nucleus then begins to indent and chromatin becomes coarser, signaling the metamyelocyte stage. In the metamyelocyte, the indentation of the nucleus is less than 50% of the hypothetical round nucleus. The cell is called a *band* when the nucleus becomes constricted without threadlike filaments, and the indentation of the nucleus is more than 50% of the hypothetical round nucleus. Finally, the cell becomes a segmented neutrophil when the nucleus becomes segmented or lobated into two to five lobes. The lobes are connected by threadlike filaments with no chromatin visible in the filament.

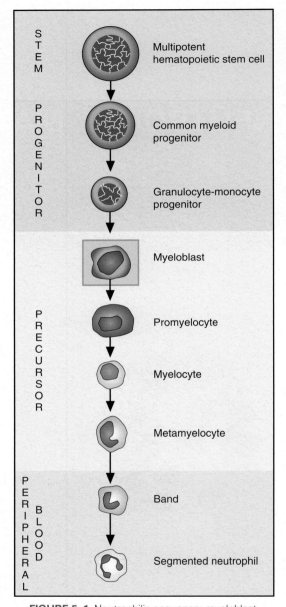

FIGURE 5–1 Neutrophilic sequence: myeloblast.

The dynamic nature of maturation is easily seen in the neutrophilic series; that is, cell maturation does not proceed in a stepwise fashion but occurs gradually from one stage to another. Thus morphologically, a cell may appear as a late promyelocyte or an early myelocyte. When there is a question of maturation stage, it is generally preferable to classify the cell at the more mature stage.

MYELOBLAST

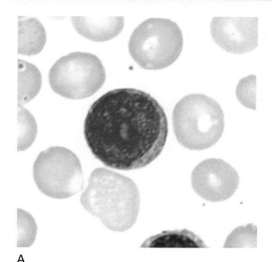

A

FIGURE 5–2A Myeloblast with no granules.

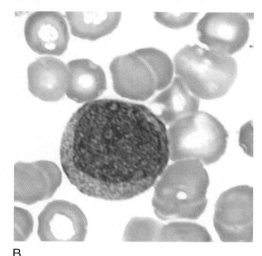

B

FIGURE 5–2B Myeloblast with up to 20 granules.

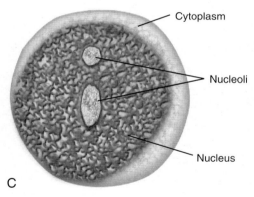

C

FIGURE 5–2C Schematic of Figure 5–2A, myeloblast.

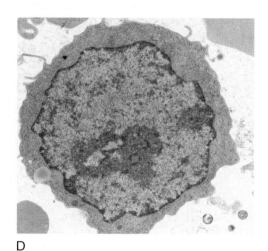

D

FIGURE 5–2D Electron micrograph of myeloblast (×16,500).

SIZE: 15 to 20 μm

NUCLEUS: Round to oval
Nucleoli: 2 to 5
Chromatin: Fine

CYTOPLASM: Moderate basophilia
Granules: Absent or up to 20

N:C RATIO: 4:1

REFERENCE INTERVAL:
Bone Marrow: 0% to 2%
Peripheral Blood: 0%

NOTE: Blasts without granulation are sometimes referred to as Type I blasts, and those with up to 20 granules as Type II blasts, although they are generally not separated as such in the differential count.

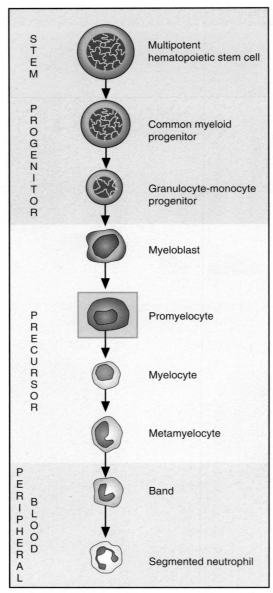

STEM

PROGENITOR

Multipotent hematopoietic stem cell

Common myeloid progenitor

Granulocyte-monocyte progenitor

Myeloblast

PRECURSOR

Promyelocyte

Myelocyte

Metamyelocyte

PERIPHERAL BLOOD

Band

Segmented neutrophil

FIGURE 5–3 Neutrophilic sequence: promyelocyte.

PROMYELOCYTE (PROGRANULOCYTE)

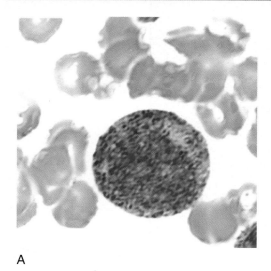

A

FIGURE 5–4A Promyelocyte.

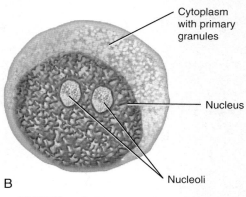

Cytoplasm
with primary
granules

Nucleus

Nucleoli

B

FIGURE 5–4B Schematic of promyelocyte.

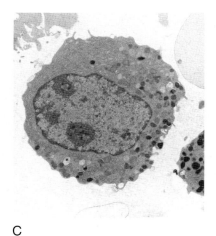

C

FIGURE 5–4C Electron micrograph of promyelocyte
(×13,000).

SIZE: 14 to 24 μm (slightly larger than myeloblast)

NUCLEUS: Round to oval
Nucleoli: 1 to 3 or more
Chromatin: Fine, but slightly coarser than
myeloblast

CYTOPLASM: Basophilic
Granules:
    PRIMARY: More than 20; may be numerous; red
        to purple or burgundy
    SECONDARY: None

N:C RATIO: 3:1

REFERENCE INTERVAL:
Bone Marrow: 2% to 5%
Peripheral Blood: 0%

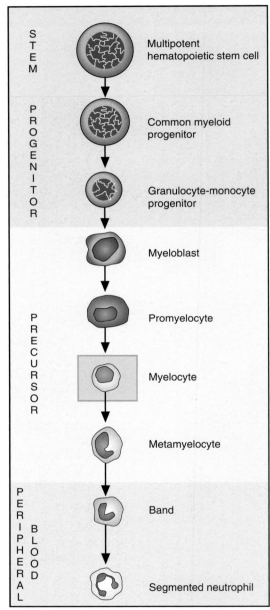

FIGURE 5–5 Neutrophilic sequence: myelocyte.

NEUTROPHILIC MYELOCYTE

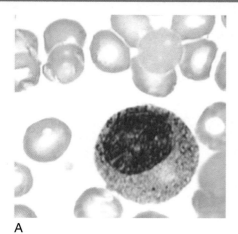

A

FIGURE 5–6A Neutrophilic myelocyte, early.

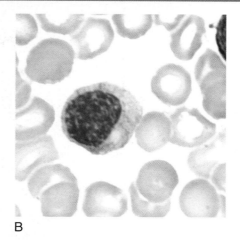

B

FIGURE 5–6B Neutrophilic myelocyte.

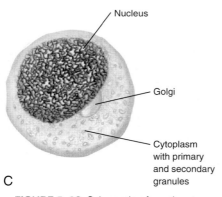

C

FIGURE 5–6C Schematic of myelocyte.

Nucleus

Golgi

Cytoplasm
with primary
and secondary
granules

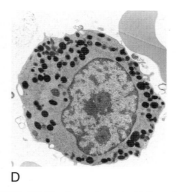

D

FIGURE 5–6D Electron micrograph of myelocyte
(×16,500).

SIZE: 12 to 18 µm

NUCLEUS: Round to oval; slightly eccentric; may have one flattened side; may have a clearing next to the
nucleus indicating the location of the Golgi
Nucleoli: Usually not visible
Chromatin: Coarse and more condensed than promyelocyte

CYTOPLASM: Slightly basophilic, to cream-colored
Granules:
PRIMARY: Few to moderate
SECONDARY: Variable number; becoming predominant as cell matures

N:C RATIO: 2:1

REFERENCE INTERVAL:
Bone Marrow: 5% to 19%
Peripheral Blood: 0%

NOTE: Secondary granules in neutrophils are too small to resolve at the light microscope level. They give the
cytoplasm a grainy or sandy appearance, and the overall color is lavender to pink. (See Figure 7–2 for
eosinophilic myelocyte.)

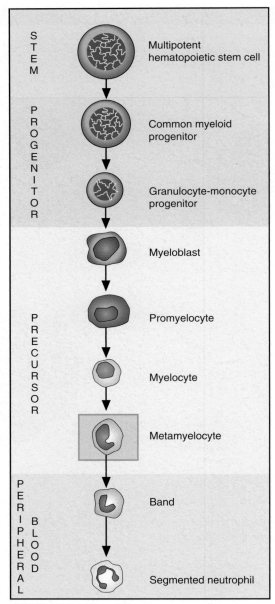

STEM

PROGENITOR

PRECURSOR

PERIPHERAL BLOOD

Multipotent hematopoietic stem cell

Common myeloid progenitor

Granulocyte-monocyte progenitor

Myeloblast

Promyelocyte

Myelocyte

Metamyelocyte

Band

Segmented neutrophil

FIGURE 5–7 Neutrophilic sequence: metamyelocyte.

NEUTROPHILIC METAMYELOCYTE

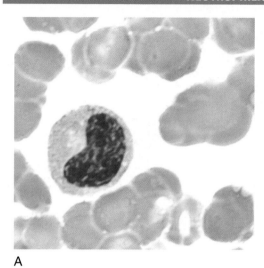

A

FIGURE 5–8A Neutrophilic metamyelocyte.

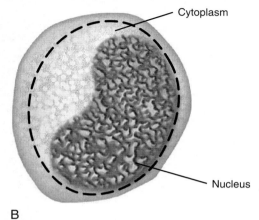

B

FIGURE 5–8B Schematic of metamyelocyte. *Dotted line* indicates hypothetical round nucleus.

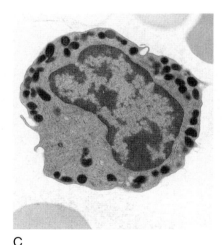

C

FIGURE 5–8C Electron micrograph of metamyelocyte (×22,250).

SIZE: 10 to 15 μm

NUCLEUS: Indented; kidney bean shape; indentation is less than 50% of the width of a hypothetical round nucleus
Nucleoli: Not visible
Chromatin: Moderately clumped

CYTOPLASM: Pale pink, to cream colored, to colorless
Granules:
   PRIMARY: Few
   SECONDARY: Many (full complement)

N:C RATIO: 1.5:1

REFERENCE INTERVAL:
Bone Marrow: 13% to 22%
Peripheral Blood: 0%

See Figure 7–4 for eosinophilic metamyelocyte.

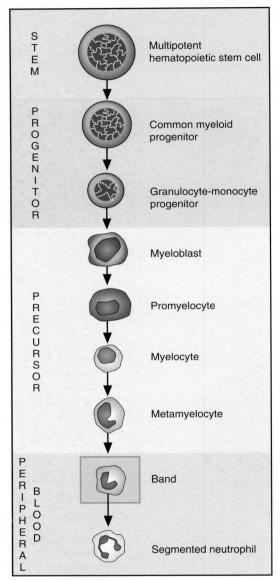

STEM

PROGENITOR

PRECURSOR

PERIPHERAL BLOOD

Multipotent hematopoietic stem cell

Common myeloid progenitor

Granulocyte-monocyte progenitor

Myeloblast

Promyelocyte

Myelocyte

Metamyelocyte

Band

Segmented neutrophil

FIGURE 5–9 Neutrophilic sequence: band.

NEUTROPHILIC BAND

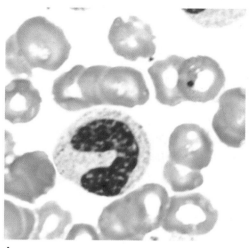

FIGURE 5–10A Neutrophilic band.

Cytoplasm

Nucleus

B

FIGURE 5–10B Schematic of band.

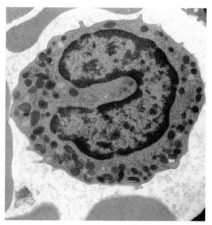

C

FIGURE 5–10C Electron micrograph of band (×22,250).

NOTE: There is so much variability in the differentiation of band neutrophils from segmented neutrophils that the College of American Pathologists does not require that they be differentiated for proficiency testing.*

SIZE: 10 to 15 μm

NUCLEUS: Constricted but no threadlike filament; indentation is more than 50% of the width of a hypothetical round nucleus

NOTE: Chromatin must be visible in constriction; may be folded over.

Nucleoli: Not visible
Chromatin: Coarse, clumped

CYTOPLASM: Pale pink, to colorless
Granules:
PRIMARY: Few
SECONDARY: Abundant

N:C RATIO: Cytoplasm predominates

REFERENCE INTERVAL:
Bone Marrow: 17% to 33%
Peripheral Blood: 0% to 5%

Refer to Table 1–1 for more examples.
See Figure 7–6 for eosinophilic band.

---

*The College of American Pathologists recommendations are available at: College of American Pathologists. Blood cell identification. In *2015 Hematology and clinical microscopy glossary*. Northfield, IL, 2015, College of American Pathologists. Available at: http://www.cap.org/ShowProperty?nodePath=/UCMCon/Contribution%20Folders/WebContent/pdf/hematology-glossary.pdf.

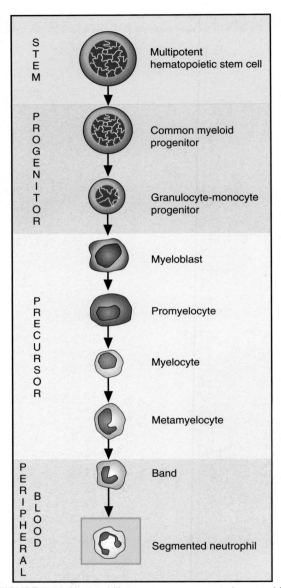

FIGURE 5–11 Neutrophilic sequence: segmented neutrophil.

SEGMENTED NEUTROPHIL
Polymorphonuclear Neutrophil

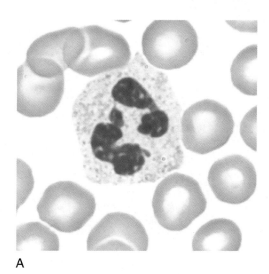

A

FIGURE 5–12A Segmented neutrophil.

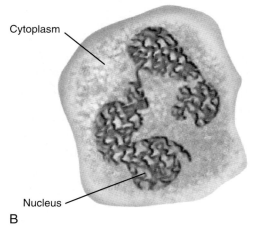

B

FIGURE 5–12B Schematic of segmented neutrophil.

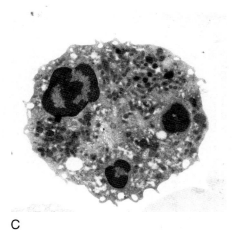

C

FIGURE 5–12C Electron micrograph of segmented neutrophil (×22,250). Specimens for electron microscopy are prepared by embedding tissue in a suitable medium, such as resin. Ultra-thin cross sections are then prepared. Because this image shows a cross section, the lobes of the nucleus appear to be separate, but are not.

SIZE: 10 to 15 μm

NUCLEUS: 2 to 5 lobes connected by thin filaments, without visible chromatin
Nucleoli: Not visible
Chromatin: Coarse, clumped

CYTOPLASM: Pale pink, cream-colored, or colorless
Granules:
PRIMARY: Rare
SECONDARY: Abundant

N:C RATIO: Cytoplasm predominates

REFERENCE INTERVAL:
Bone Marrow: 3% to 11%
Peripheral Blood: 50% to 70%

Refer to Table 1–1 for more examples.

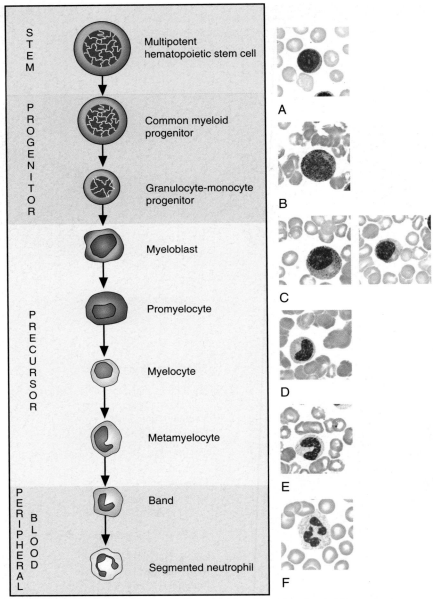

FIGURE 5–13 Neutrophilic sequence with **A**, myeloblast; **B**, promyelocyte; **C**, myelocyte; **D**, metamyelocyte; **E**, band; **F**, segmented neutrophil.

CHAPTER 6

MONOCYTE MATURATION

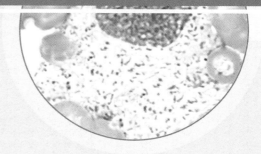

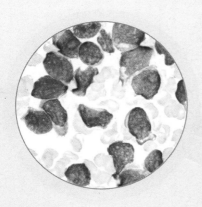

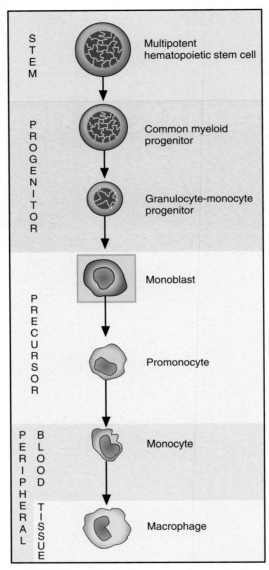

FIGURE 6–1 Monocyte sequence—monoblast.

All photomicrographs are × 1000 original magnification with Wright-Giemsa staining unless stated otherwise.

MONOBLAST

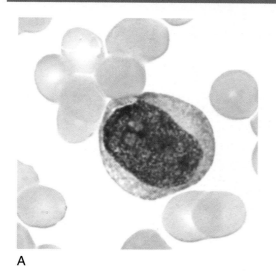

A

FIGURE 6–2A Monoblast.

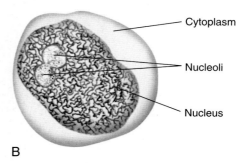

B

FIGURE 6–2B Schematic of monoblast.

SIZE: 12 to 18 μm

NUCLEUS: Round to oval; may be irregularly shaped
Nucleoli: 1 to 2; may not be visible
Chromatin: Fine

CYTOPLASM: Light blue to gray
Granules: None

N:C RATIO: 4:1

REFERENCE INTERVAL:
Bone Marrow: Not defined
Peripheral Blood: 0%

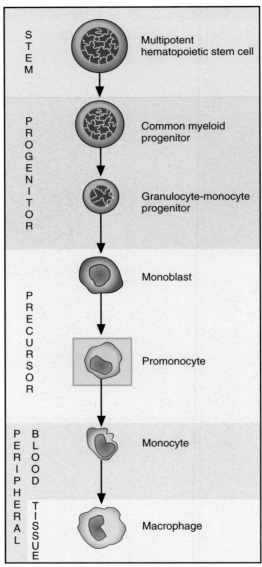

FIGURE 6–3 Monocyte sequence—promonocyte.

PROMONOCYTE

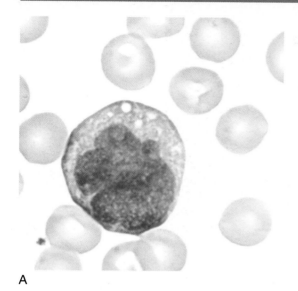

A

FIGURE 6–4A Promonocyte.

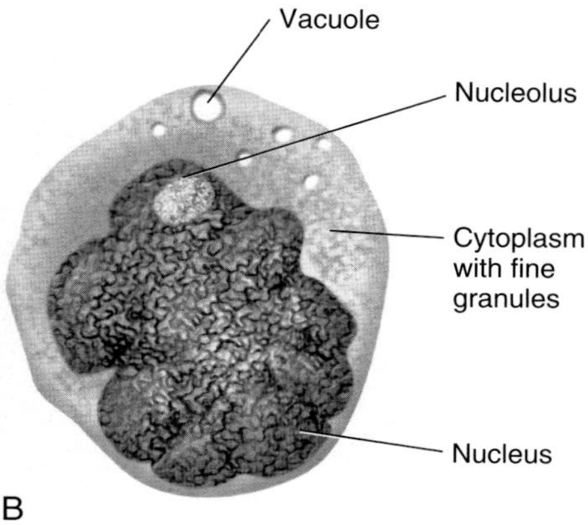

Vacuole

Nucleolus

Cytoplasm with fine granules

Nucleus

B

FIGURE 6–4B Schematic of promonocyte.

SIZE: 12 to 20 μm

NUCLEUS: Irregularly shaped; folded; may have brainlike convolutions
Nucleoli: May or may not be visible
Chromatin: Fine to lacy

CYTOPLASM: Light blue to gray
Granules: Fine azurophilic (burgundy colored)

N:C RATIO: 2 to 3:1

REFERENCE INTERVAL:
Bone Marrow: Less than 1%
Peripheral Blood: 0%

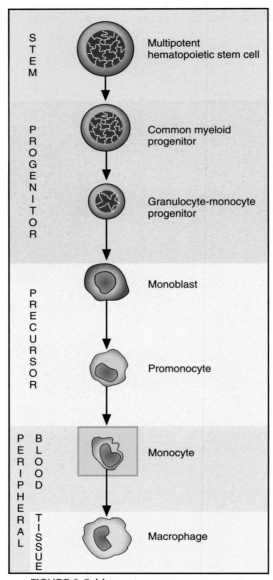

STEM

PROGENITOR

PRECURSOR

PERIPHERAL BLOOD

TISSUE

Multipotent hematopoietic stem cell

Common myeloid progenitor

Granulocyte-monocyte progenitor

Monoblast

Promonocyte

Monocyte

Macrophage

FIGURE 6–5 Monocyte sequence: monocyte.

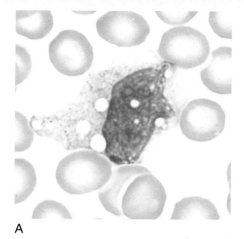

A

FIGURE 6–6A Monocyte.

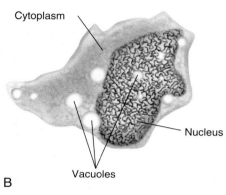

Cytoplasm

Nucleus

Vacuoles

B

FIGURE 6–6B Schematic of monocyte.

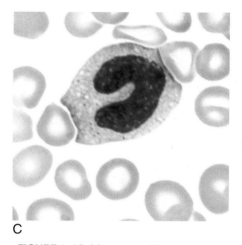

C

FIGURE 6–6C Monocyte without vacuoles.

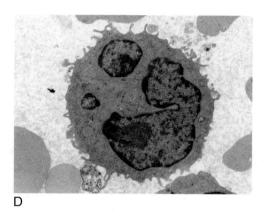

D

FIGURE 6–6D Electron micrograph of monocyte (×16,500). Specimens for electron microscopy are prepared by embedding tissue in a suitable medium, such as resin. Ultra-thin cross sections are then prepared. Because this image shows a cross section, the lobes of the nucleus appear to be separate, but are not.

SIZE: 12 to 20 μm

NUCLEUS: Variable; may be round, horseshoe shaped, or kidney shaped; often has folds producing brainlike convolutions
Nucleoli: Not visible
Chromatin: Lacy

CYTOPLASM: Blue-gray; may have pseudopods
Granules: Many fine granules frequently giving the appearance of ground glass
Vacuoles: Absent to numerous

N:C RATIO: Variable

REFERENCE INTERVAL:
Bone Marrow: 2%
Peripheral Blood: 3% to 11%
Refer to Table 1-1 for more examples.

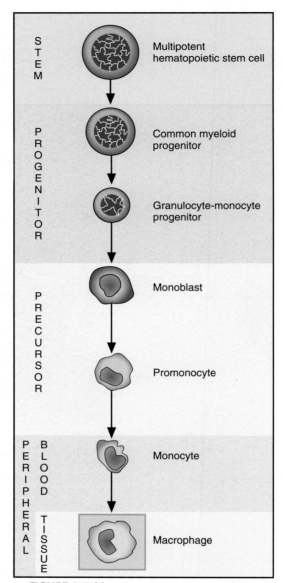

FIGURE 6–7 Monocyte sequence: macrophage.

MACROPHAGE (HISTIOCYTE)

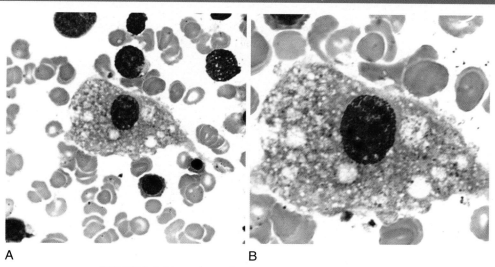

A B

FIGURE 6–8 Macrophage. Bone marrow **A**, ×500; **B**, ×1000.

SIZE: 15 to 80 μm

NUCLEUS: Eccentric, kidney or egg-shaped, indented, or elongated
Nucleoli: 1 to 2
Chromatin: Fine, dispersed

CYTOPLASM: Abundant with irregular borders; may contain ingested material
Granules: Many coarse azurophilic (burgundy-colored)
Vacuoles: May be present

REFERENCE INTERVAL: Macrophages reside in tissues such as bone marrow, spleen, liver, lungs, and others. Rarely, seen in the peripheral blood during severe sepsis.

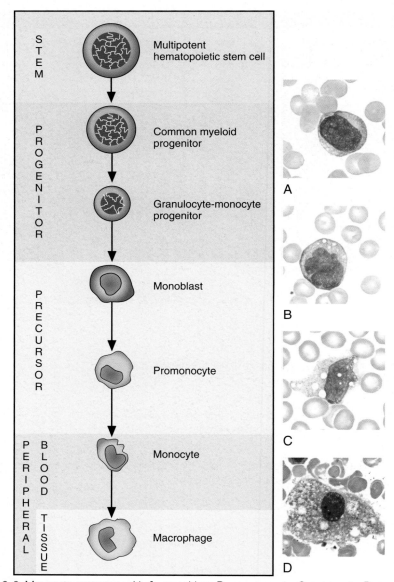

FIGURE 6–9 Monocyte sequence with **A**, monoblast; **B**, promonocyte; **C**, monocyte; **D**. macrophage.

CHAPTER 7

EOSINOPHIL MATURATION

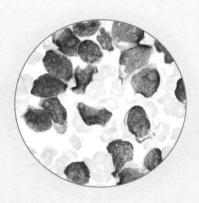

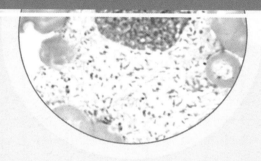

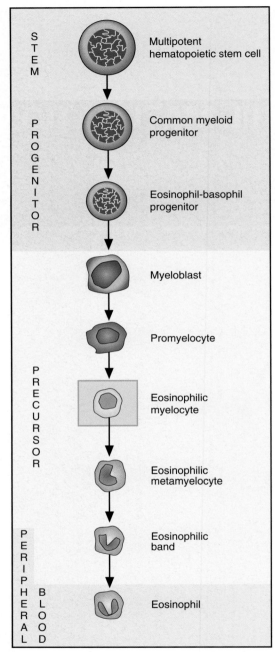

FIGURE 7–1 Eosinophilic sequence: eosinophilic myelocyte.

All photomicrographs are × 1000 original magnification with Wright–Giemsa staining unless stated otherwise.

EOSINOPHILIC MYELOCYTE

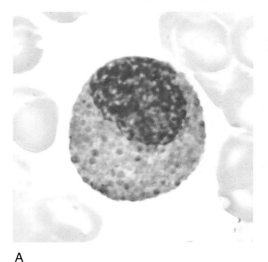

A

FIGURE 7–2A Eosinophilic myelocyte.

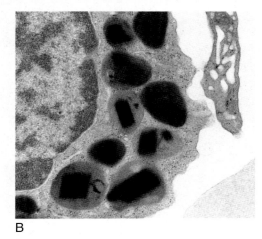

B

FIGURE 7–2B Electron micrograph of eosinophilic granules to demonstrate crystalline structure of granules.

SIZE: 12 to 18 μm

NUCLEUS: Round to oval; may have one flattened side
Nucleoli: Usually not visible
Chromatin: Coarse and more condensed than promyelocyte

CYTOPLASM: Colorless to pink
Granules:
 PRIMARY: Few to moderate
 SECONDARY: Variable number; pale orange to dark orange; round; appear refractile

N:C RATIO: 2:1 to 1:1

REFERENCE INTERVAL:
Bone Marrow: 0% to 2%
Peripheral Blood: 0%

 NOTE: This chapter begins with the image of the myelocyte, rather than the blast, because it is at the myelocyte stage that secondary granules, which define a cell as an eosinophil, first appear.

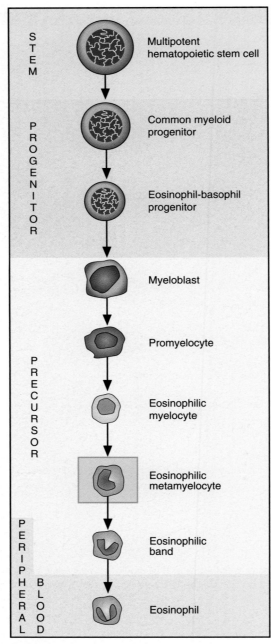

FIGURE 7–3 Eosinophilic sequence: eosinophilic metamyelocyte.

EOSINOPHILIC METAMYELOCYTE

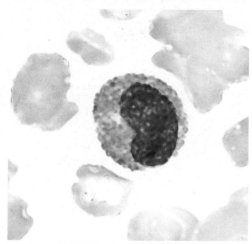

FIGURE 7–4 Eosinophilic metamyelocyte.

SIZE: 10 to 15 µm

NUCLEUS: Indented; kidney bean shape; indentation is less than 50% of the width of the hypothetical round nucleus
Nucleoli: Not visible
Chromatin: Coarse, clumped

CYTOPLASM: Colorless, cream-colored
Granules:
PRIMARY: Few
SECONDARY: Many pale orange to dark orange; appear refractile

N:C RATIO: 1.5:1

REFERENCE INTERVAL:
Bone Marrow: 0% to 2%
Peripheral Blood: 0%

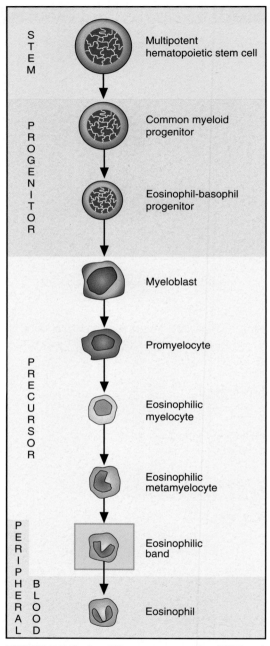

FIGURE 7–5 Eosinophilic sequence: eosinophilic band.

EOSINOPHILIC BAND

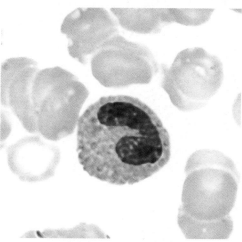

FIGURE 7–6 Eosinophilic band.

SIZE: 10 to 15 μm

NUCLEUS: Constricted but no threadlike filament; indentation is more than 50% of the width of a hypothetical round nucleus

NOTE: Chromatin must be visible in constriction.

Nucleoli: Not visible
Chromatin: Coarse, clumped

CYTOPLASM: Colorless, cream-colored
Granules:
PRIMARY: Few
SECONDARY: Abundant pale to dark orange; appear refractile

N:C RATIO: Cytoplasm predominates

REFERENCE INTERVAL:
Bone Marrow: 0% to 2%
Peripheral Blood: Rarely seen

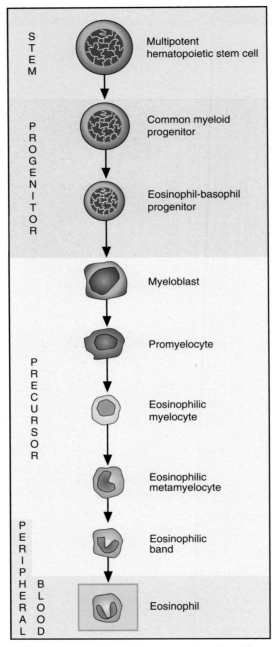

FIGURE 7–7 Eosinophilic sequence: eosinophil.

EOSINOPHIL

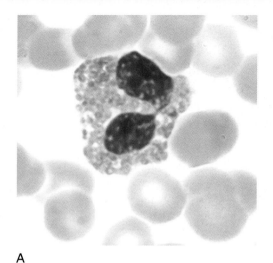

A

FIGURE 7–8A Eosinophil.

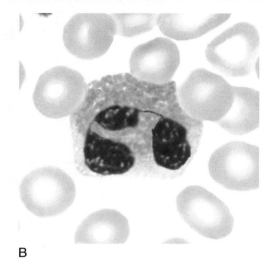

B

FIGURE 7–8B Eosinophil with 3 lobes.

SIZE: 12 to 17 μm

NUCLEUS: Two to three lobes connected by thin filaments without visible chromatin; majority of mature cells have two lobes
Nucleoli: Not visible
Chromatin: Coarse, clumped

CYTOPLASM: Cream-colored; may have irregular borders
Granules:
   PRIMARY: Rare
   SECONDARY: Abundant pale orange to dark orange; appear refractile

N:C RATIO: Cytoplasm predominates

REFERENCE INTERVAL:
Bone Marrow: 0% to 3%
Peripheral Blood: 0% to 5%
   Refer to Table 1-1 for more examples.

   NOTE: Eosinophils are fragile and may easily fracture when preparing blood film.

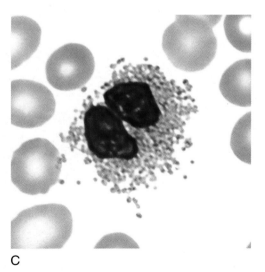

C

FIGURE 7–8C Fractured eosinophil.

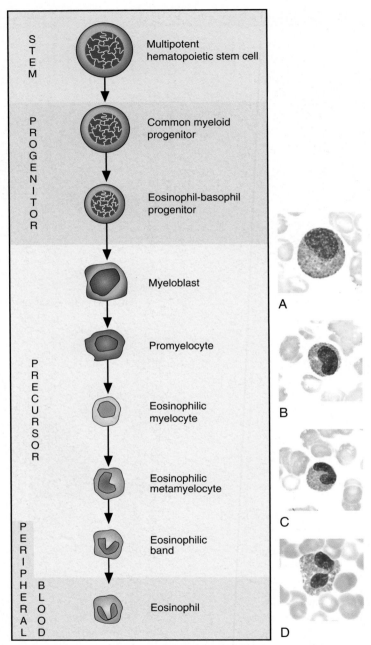

FIGURE 7–9 Eosinophilic sequence with **A**, eosinophilic myelocyte; **B**, eosinophilic metamyelocyte; **C**, eosinophilic band; **D**, eosinophil.

CHAPTER 8

BASOPHIL MATURATION

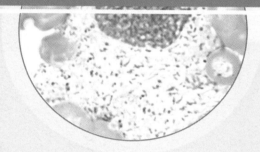

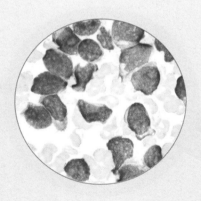

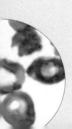

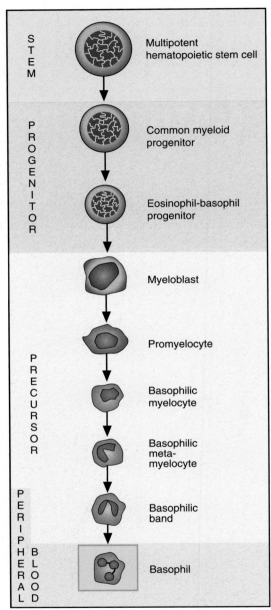

FIGURE 8–1 Basophilic sequence: Basophil. Maturation parallels that of the neutrophil; however, immature stages are very rare and generally seen only in basophil proliferative disorders.

All photomicrographs are × 1000 original magnification with Wright-Giemsa staining unless stated otherwise.

BASOPHIL

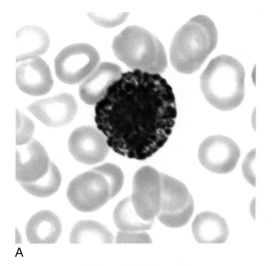

A

FIGURE 8–2A Basophil.

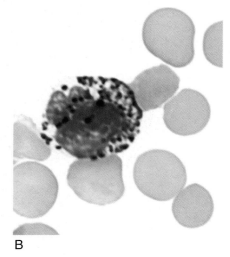

B

FIGURE 8–2B Basophil. Note that granules are water-soluble and may be dissolved during the staining process, leaving clear areas in the cytoplasm.

SIZE: 10-14 μm

NUCLEUS: Usually two lobes connected by thin filaments without visible chromatin
Nucleoli: Not visible
Chromatin: Coarse, clumped

CYTOPLASM: Lavender to colorless
Granules:
PRIMARY: Rare
SECONDARY: Large, variable in number with uneven distribution, may obscure nucleus (Figure 8–2, *A*); deep purple to black; irregularly shaped. Granules are water-soluble and may be washed out during staining; thus they appear as empty areas in the cytoplasm (Figure 8–2, *B*).

N:C RATIO: Cytoplasm predominates

REFERENCE INTERVAL:
Bone Marrow: Less than 1%
Peripheral Blood: 0% to 1%

Refer to Table 1-1 for more examples.

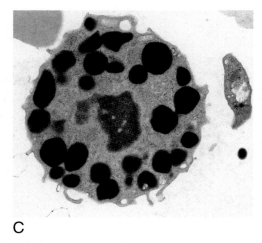

C

FIGURE 8–2C Electron micrograph of basophil (×28,750).

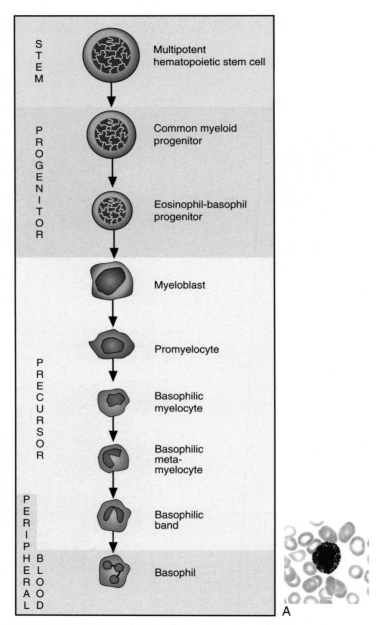

FIGURE 8–3 Maturation parallels that of the neutrophil; however, immature stages are very rare and generally seen only in basophil proliferative disorders. **A**, Basophil.

CHAPTER 9

LYMPHOCYTE MATURATION

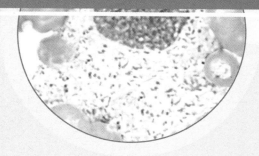

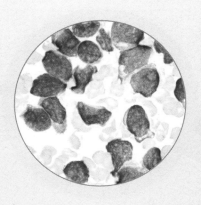

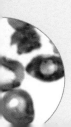

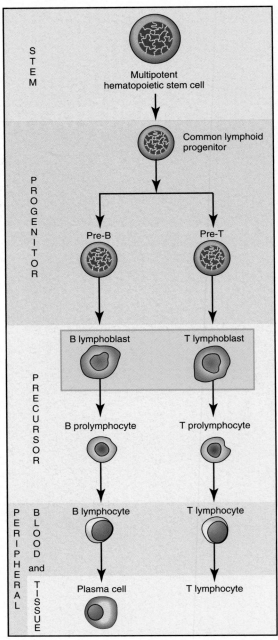

FIGURE 9–1 Lymphocyte sequence: B and T lymphoblasts.

All photomicrographs are ×1000 original magnification with Wright-Giemsa staining unless stated otherwise.

LYMPHOBLAST

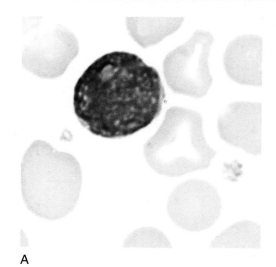

A

FIGURE 9–2A Lymphoblast.

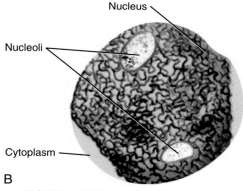

Nucleus

Nucleoli

Cytoplasm

B

FIGURE 9–2B Schematic of lymphoblast.

SIZE: 10 to 20 μm

NUCLEUS: Round to oval
Nucleoli: Greater than or equal to 1
Chromatin: Fine, evenly stained

CYTOPLASM: Scant; slightly to moderately
   basophilic
Granules: None

N:C RATIO: 7:1 to 4:1

REFERENCE INTERVAL:
Bone Marrow: Not defined
Peripheral Blood: 0%

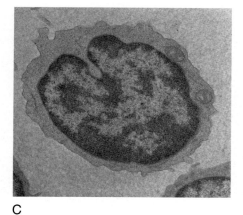

C

FIGURE 9–2C Electron micrograph of lymphoblast
(×28,750). Lymphoblasts are difficult to distinguish
morphologically in normal bone marrow.

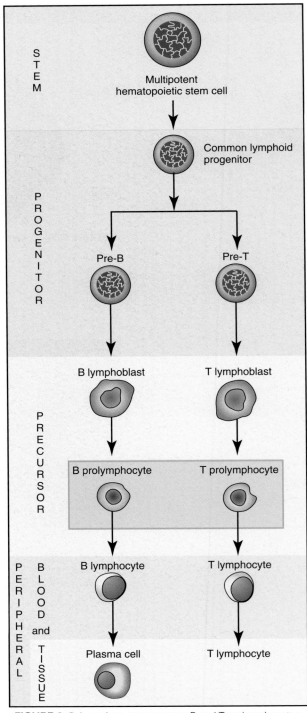

FIGURE 9–3 Lymphocyte sequence: B and T prolymphocytes.

PROLYMPHOCYTE

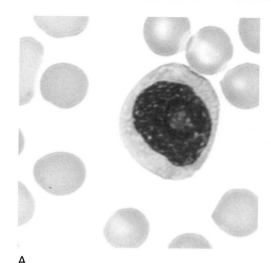

A

FIGURE 9–4A Prolymphocyte. Prolymphocytes are difficult to distinguish morphologically in normal bone marrow

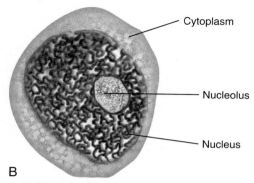

B

FIGURE 9–4B Schematic of prolymphocyte.

SIZE: 9 to 18 µm

NUCLEUS: Round or indented
Nucleoli: 0 to 1; usually single, prominent, large nucleolus
Chromatin: Slightly clumped; intermediate between lymphoblast and mature lymphocyte

CYTOPLASM: Light blue
Granules: None

N:C RATIO: 3 to 4:1

REFERENCE INTERVAL:
Bone Marrow: Not defined
Peripheral Blood: None

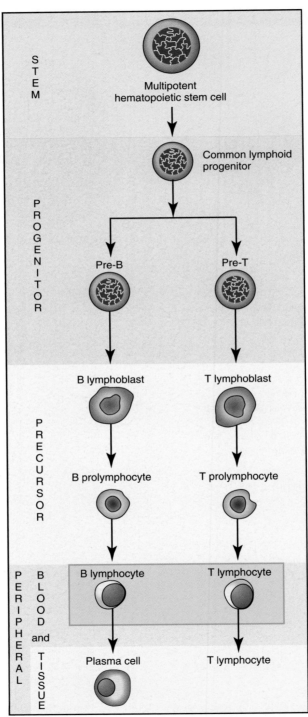

FIGURE 9–5 Lymphocyte sequence: B and T lymphocytes. (NOTE: T lymphocytes cannot be distinguished from B lymphocytes with Wright stain.)

LYMPHOCYTE

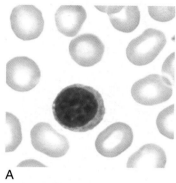

FIGURE 9–6A Small lymphocyte.

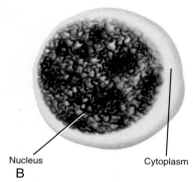

Nucleus   Cytoplasm

B

FIGURE 9–6B Schematic of lymphocyte.

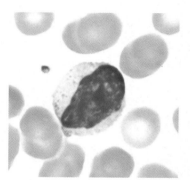

C

FIGURE 9–6C Large lymphocyte with irregular nucleus and more abundant cytoplasm than small lymphocyte.

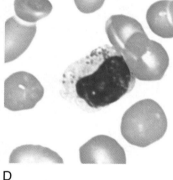

D

FIGURE 9–6D Large granular lymphocyte with prominent azurophilic granules in cytoplasm.

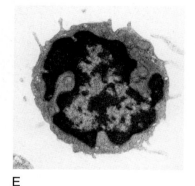

E

FIGURE 9–6E Electron micrograph of lymphocyte (×30,000).

SIZE: 7 to 18 μm

NUCLEUS: Round to oval; may be slightly indented
Nucleoli: Occasional
Chromatin: Condensed, clumped, blocky, smudged

CYTOPLASM: Scant to moderate; sky blue; vacuoles may be present
Granules: None in a small lymphocyte; may be a few azurophilic in larger lymphocytes; if granules are prominent, the cell is called a large granular lymphocyte.

N:C RATIO: 5:1 to 2:1

REFERENCE INTERVAL (FOR COMBINED SMALL AND LARGE LYMPHOCYTES):
Bone Marrow: 5% to 15%
Peripheral Blood: 20% to 40%

Refer to Table 1–1 for more examples.
Refer to Appendix Table A–1 for a comparison of myelocytes and lymphocytes.

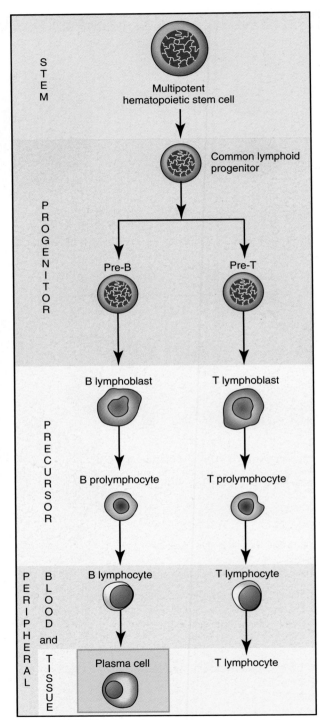

FIGURE 9–7 Lymphocyte sequence: plasma cell.

PLASMA CELL

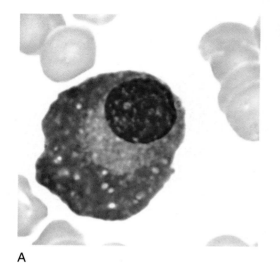

A

FIGURE 9–8A Plasma cell.

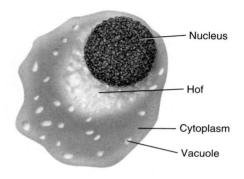

B

FIGURE 9–8B Schematic of plasma cell.

Nucleus

Hof

Cytoplasm

Vacuole

SIZE: 8 to 20 μm

NUCLEUS: Round or oval; eccentric
Nucleoli: None
Chromatin: Coarse

CYTOPLASM: Deeply basophilic, often with perinuclear clear zone (hof)
Granules: None
Vacuoles: None to several

N:C RATIO: 2:1 to 1:1

REFERENCE INTERVAL:
Bone Marrow: 0% to 1%
Peripheral Blood: 0%

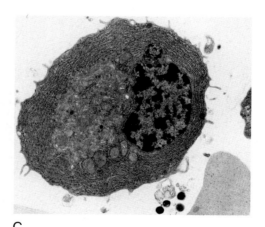

C

FIGURE 9–8C Electron micrograph of plasma cell (×17,500).

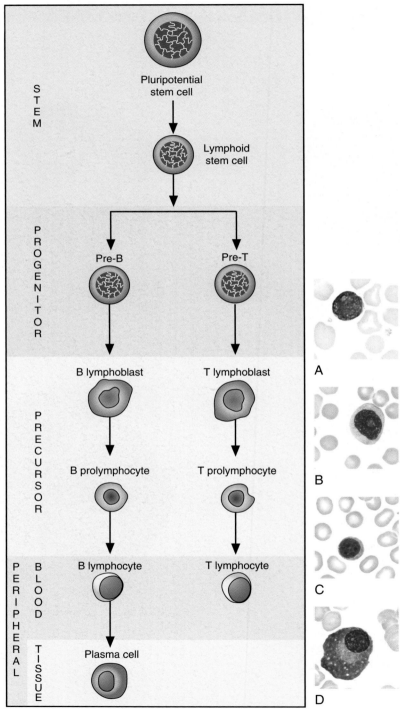

FIGURE 9–9 Lymphocyte sequence with **A**, lymphoblast; **B**, prolymphocyte; **C**, lymphocyte; **D**, plasma cell.

CHAPTER 10

VARIATIONS IN SIZE AND COLOR OF ERYTHROCYTES

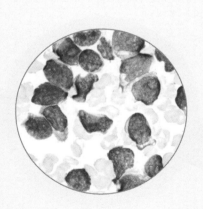

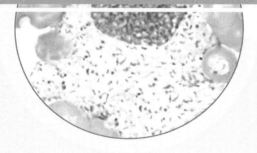

VARIATIONS IN SIZE

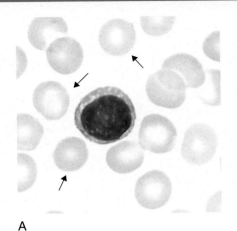

A

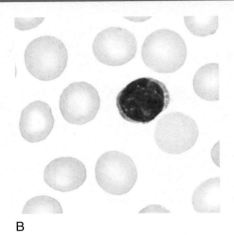

B

FIGURE 10–1A Microcytes (mean cell volume [MCV] <80 fL).

ASSOCIATED WITH: Iron deficiency anemia, thalassemia minor, chronic inflammation (some cases), lead poisoning, hemoglobinopathies (some), sideroblastic anemia

FIGURE 10–1B Normocytes (mean cell volume [MCV] 80-100 fL).

Normal erythrocytes are approximately the same size as the nucleus of a small lymphocyte.

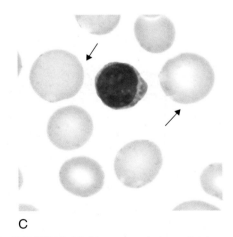

C

FIGURE 10–1C Macrocytes (mean cell volume [MCV] >100 fL).

ASSOCIATED WITH: Liver disease, vitamin B_{12} deficiency, folate deficiency, neonates, reticulocytosis

Anisocytosis is the variation in red blood cell (RBC) diameter (or RBC volume) on a blood film. This variation correlates with the electronically determined red blood cell distribution width (RDW). An RDW greater than 14.5% indicates a heterogeneous population of RBCs, and a variety of sizes of RBCs should be seen. A low RDW is of no significance.

ANISOCYTOSIS

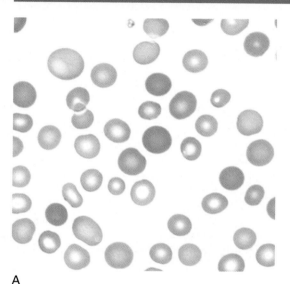

A

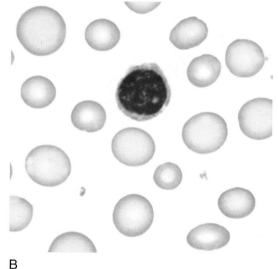

B

FIGURE 10–2A Heterogeneous population of erythrocytes, indicating anisocytosis (red blood cell distribution width [RDW] >14.5%). (x500)

FIGURE 10–2B When two distinct populations of RBCs are seen, it is termed a *dimorphic population* (red blood cell distribution width [RDW] >14.5%).

ASSOCIATED WITH: Anemias; especially iron deficiency, megaloblastic, and hemolytic

ASSOCIATED WITH: Transfusion; myelodysplastic syndromes; sideroblastic anemia; vitamin B_{12}, folate, or iron deficiency: early in treatment process

VARIATION IN COLOR OF ERYTHROCYTES

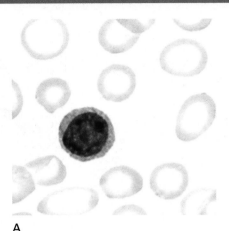

A

FIGURE 10–3A Hypochromia. The central pallor zone of the erythrocyte must be greater than one-third of the diameter of the cell before it is classified as hypochromic. (Note: the mean cell hemoglobin concentration [MCHC], not the mean cell hemoglobin [MCH], should be used as a gauge of hypochromia; however, the MCHC is not always decreased when few hypochromic cells are seen.)

     ASSOCIATED WITH: Iron deficiency anemia, thalassemias, sideroblastic anemia, lead poisoning, some cases of anemia of chronic inflammation

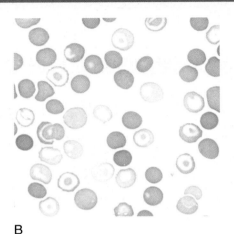

B

FIGURE 10–3B Dichromic population of erythrocytes (PB × 500). Two populations of red blood cells (RBCs) are shown: one normochromic and one hypochromic.

ASSOCIATED WITH: Transfusions, sideroblastic anemia

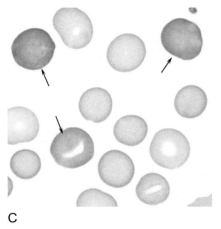

C

FIGURE 10–3C Polychromasia; retained ribonucleic acid (RNA) in RBCs.

     ASSOCIATED WITH: Acute and chronic hemorrhage, hemolysis, effective treatment for anemia, neonates

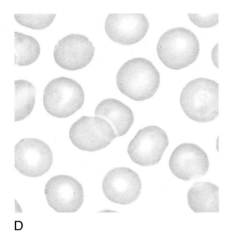

D

FIGURE 10–3D Normochromic erythrocytes. (MCHC 32-36 g/dL or 32%-36%.) For comparison with hypochromic and polychromatic erythrocytes.

CHAPTER 11

VARIATIONS IN SHAPE AND DISTRIBUTION OF ERYTHROCYTES

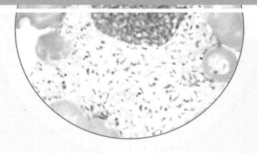

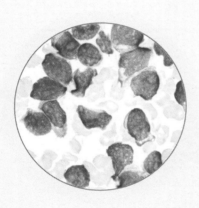

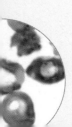

POIKILOCYTOSIS

Poikilocytosis is a general term for the presence of abnormally shaped red blood cells. In most cases, we have opted to use the more specific name for each abnormally shaped red blood cell in place of the term *poikilocytosis*.

ACANTHOCYTE
Spur Cell

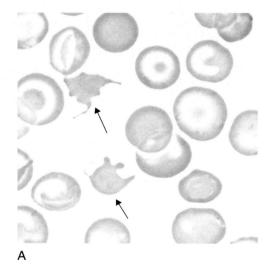

A

FIGURE 11–1A Acanthocytes.

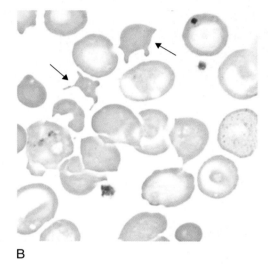

B

FIGURE 11–1B Acanthocytes.

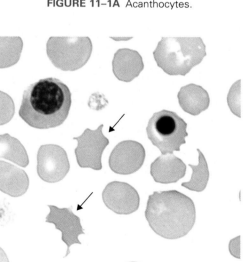

C

FIGURE 11–1C Acanthocytes; two nucleated red blood cells in field.

DESCRIPTION: Dark red to salmon, lacking central pallor. Erythrocyte with multiple irregularly spaced projections often with drumstick ends, varying in width, length, and number

ASSOCIATED WITH: Severe liver disease, splenectomy, malabsorption, hypothyroidism, vitamin E deficiency, abetalipoproteinemia

SCHISTOCYTE
Red Blood Cell Fragments

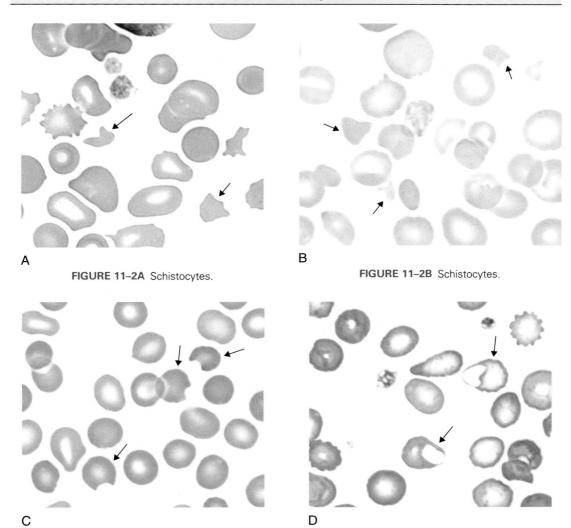

A

FIGURE 11–2A Schistocytes.

B

FIGURE 11–2B Schistocytes.

C

FIGURE 11–2C Bite cells.

D

FIGURE 11–2D Blister cells.

DESCRIPTION: Red to salmon. Fragmented erythrocytes; many sizes and shapes may be present on a smear; often display pointed extremities

ASSOCIATED WITH: Microangiopathic hemolytic anemia (hemolytic uremic syndrome, thrombotic thrombocytopenic purpura, disseminated intravascular coagulation), severe burns, renal graft rejection

NOTE: Bite and blister cells are the result of splenic pitting of Heinz bodies (see Figure 12-5, B). These cells are often included in the schistocyte category.

ECHINOCYTE
Burr Cell

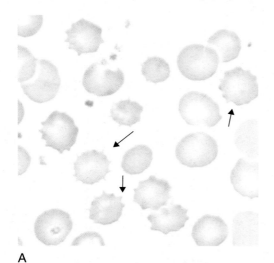

A

FIGURE 11–3A Echinocytes/burr cells.

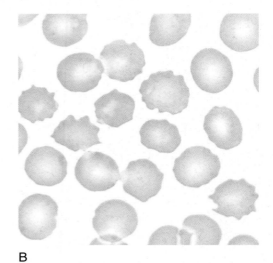

B

FIGURE 11–3B Echinocytes/burr cells.

DESCRIPTION: Erythrocyte with short, evenly spaced projections usually with central pallor

ASSOCIATED WITH: Uremia, pyruvate kinase deficiency, microangiopathic hemolytic anemia, neonates (especially premature), artifact

SPHEROCYTE

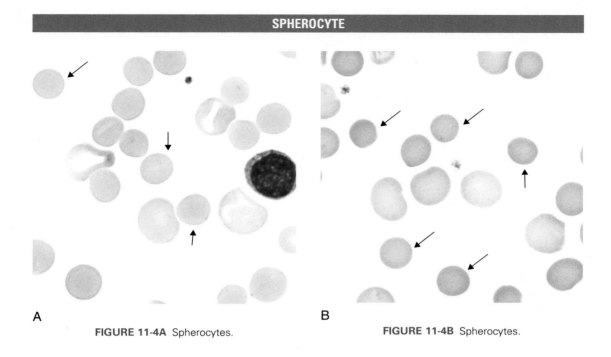

A

FIGURE 11-4A Spherocytes.

B

FIGURE 11-4B Spherocytes.

DESCRIPTION: Round; no central pallor zone. Darker than surrounding red blood cells

ASSOCIATED WITH: Hereditary spherocytosis, some hemolytic anemias, transfused cells, severe burns

TARGET CELL
Codocyte

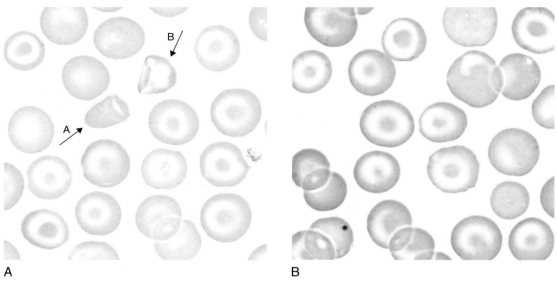

A

B

FIGURE 11-5A Target cells.   **FIGURE 11-5B** Target cells.

DESCRIPTION: Red to salmon; bull's eye; central concentration of hemoglobin surrounded by colorless area with peripheral ring of hemoglobin resembling bull's eye; may be bell (Figure 11-5, *A, arrow A*) or cup (see Figure 11-5, *A, arrow B*) shaped.

ASSOCIATED WITH: Hemoglobinopathies, thalassemia, iron deficiency anemia, splenectomy, obstructive liver disease

SICKLE CELL
Drepanocyte

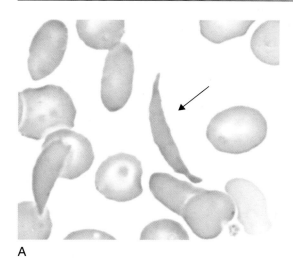

A

FIGURE 11–6A Sickle cells.

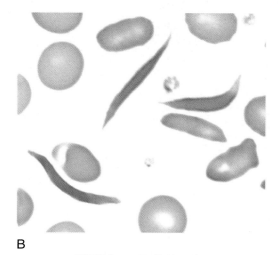

B

FIGURE 11–6B Sickle cells.

DESCRIPTION: Dark red to salmon, lacks central pallor. Elongated cell with point on each end; may be curved or S-shaped. Composed of hemoglobin S polymers

ASSOCIATED WITH: Homozygous hemoglobin S disease, sometimes hemoglobin SC disease

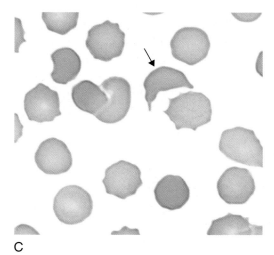

C

FIGURE 11–6C Schistocyte resembling sickle cell. (Note: Central area is markedly thicker than the ends.)

HEMOGLOBIN C CRYSTAL

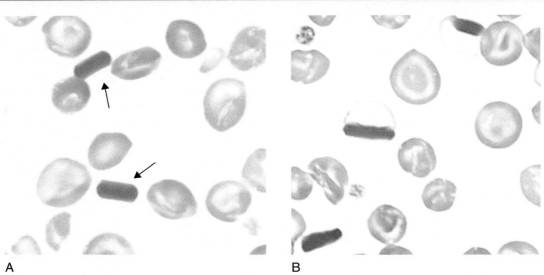

A

FIGURE 11–7A Hemoglobin CC crystals.

B

FIGURE 11–7B Hemoglobin CC crystals with visible red blood cell membrane.

DESCRIPTION: Dark red, hexagonal; usually one crystal per cell; composed of hemoglobin C

ASSOCIATED WITH: Homozygous hemoglobin C disease

HEMOGLOBIN SC CRYSTAL

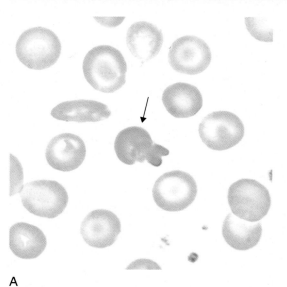

A

FIGURE 11–8A Hemoglobin SC.

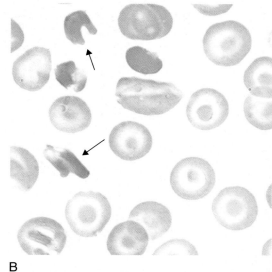

B

FIGURE 11–8B Hemoglobin SC.

DESCRIPTION: Dark red; 1 to 2 fingerlike projections; may look like a mitten or the Washington Monument (obelisk); cell may appear folded; 1 to 2 per cell; composed of hemoglobin SC

ASSOCIATED WITH: Hemoglobin SC disease

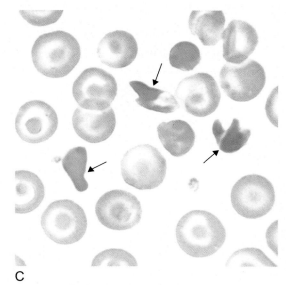

C

FIGURE 11–8C Hemoglobin SC.

ELLIPTOCYTE/OVALOCYTE

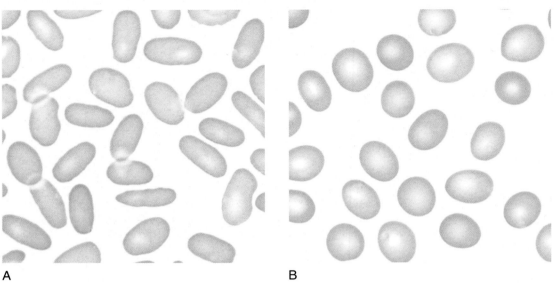

A

FIGURE 11–9A Elliptocytes.

B

FIGURE 11–9B Ovalocytes.

DESCRIPTION: Elliptocyte: cigar-shaped erythrocyte

DESCRIPTION: Ovalocyte: egg-shaped erythrocyte

ASSOCIATED WITH: Hereditary elliptocytosis or ovalocytosis, thalassemia major, iron deficiency anemia, megaloblastic anemias (macro-ovalocytes), myelophthisic anemias

TEARDROP CELL
Dacryocyte

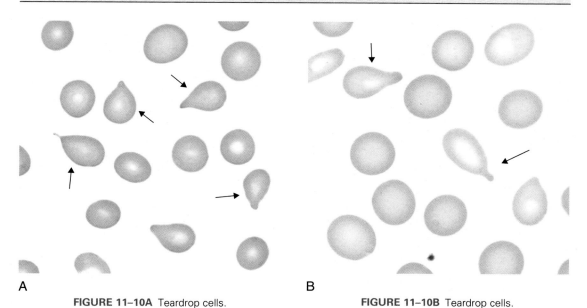

FIGURE 11–10A Teardrop cells.

FIGURE 11–10B Teardrop cells.

DESCRIPTION: Erythrocyte shaped like a teardrop or pear; may have one blunt projection

ASSOCIATED WITH: Primary myelofibrosis, thalassemia, myelophthisic anemia, other causes of extramedullary hematopoiesis

STOMATOCYTE

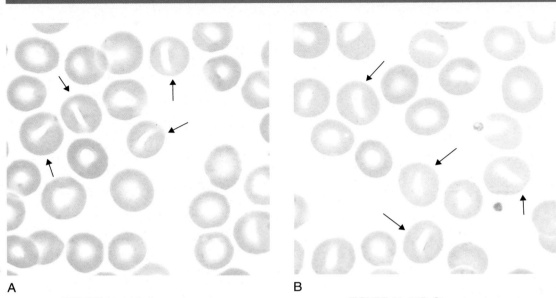

A

FIGURE 11–11A Stomatocytes.

B

FIGURE 11–11B Stomatocytes.

DESCRIPTION: Erythrocyte with slitlike area of central pallor (similar to a mouth or stoma)

ASSOCIATED WITH: Hereditary stomatocytosis, alcoholism, liver disease, Rh null phenotype, artifact

DISTRIBUTION
ROULEAUX

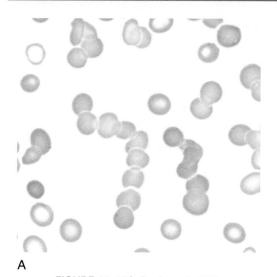

A

FIGURE 11–12A Rouleaux (×500).

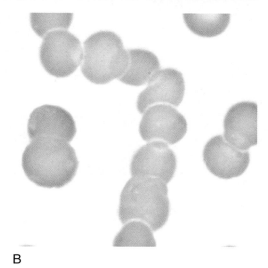

B

FIGURE 11–12B Rouleaux (×1000).

DESCRIPTION: Erythrocytes arranged in rows like stacks of coins; increased proteins in patients with rouleaux may make the background of the slide appear blue

ASSOCIATED WITH: Acute and chronic inflammatory disorders, plasma cell myeloma, lymphoplasmacytic lymphoma

NOTE: The aggregates will disperse with saline.

AUTOAGGLUTINATION

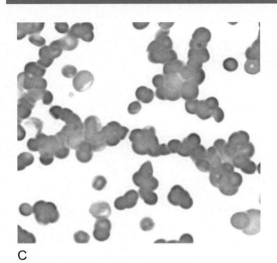

C

FIGURE 11–12C Autoagglutination (×500).

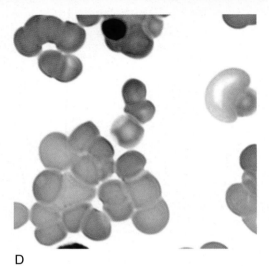

D

FIGURE 11–12D Autoagglutination (×1000).

DESCRIPTION: Clumping of erythrocytes; outlines of individual cells may not be evident

ASSOCIATED WITH: Antigen-antibody reactions

NOTE: The Aggregates will not disperse with saline.

CHAPTER 12

INCLUSIONS IN ERYTHROCYTES

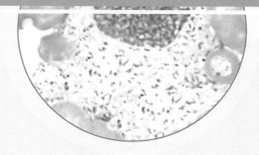

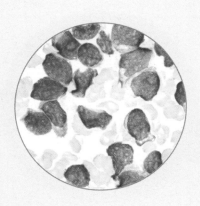

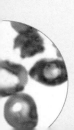

HOWELL-JOLLY BODIES

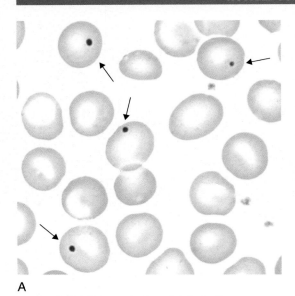

A

FIGURE 12–1A Howell-Jolly bodies.

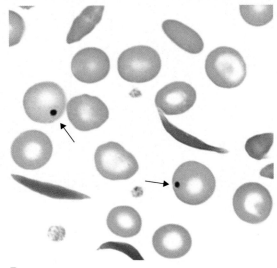

B

FIGURE 12–1B Howell-Jolly bodies in a patient with sickle cell anemia.

COLOR: Dark blue to purple

SHAPE: Round to oval

SIZE: 0.5 to 1.5 μm

NUMBER PER CELL: Usually 1; may be multiple

COMPOSITION: DNA (deoxyribonucleic acid)

ASSOCIATED WITH: Splenectomy, hyposplenism, megaloblastic anemia, hemolytic anemia

BASOPHILIC STIPPLING

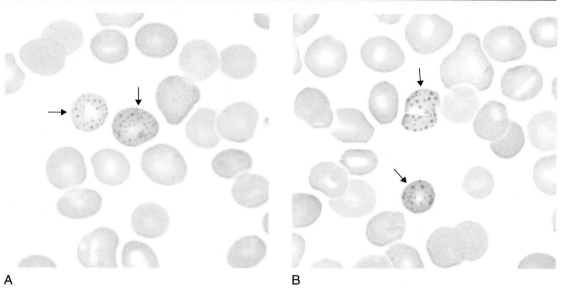

A

FIGURE 12–2A Basophilic stippling.

B

FIGURE 12–2B Basophilic stippling.

COLOR: Dark blue to purple

SHAPE: Fine or coarse punctate granules

NUMBER PER CELL: Numerous with fairly even distribution

COMPOSITION: RNA (ribonucleic acid)

ASSOCIATED WITH: Lead intoxication, thalassemia, abnormal heme synthesis

PAPPENHEIMER BODIES
Siderotic Granules

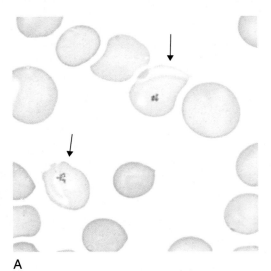

A

FIGURE 12–3A Pappenheimer bodies (Wright stain).

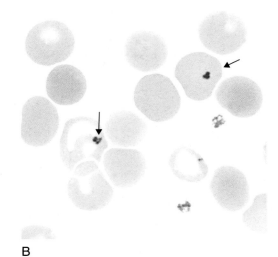

B

FIGURE 12–3B Pappenheimer bodies (Wright stain).

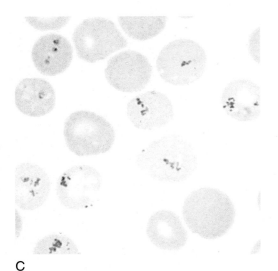

C

FIGURE 12–3C Siderotic granules (iron stain).

COLOR: Light blue

SHAPE: Fine irregular granules in clusters

NUMBER PER CELL: Usually one cluster; may be multiples; often at periphery of cell

COMPOSITION: Iron

ASSOCIATED WITH: Splenectomy, hemolytic anemia, sideroblastic anemia, megaloblastic anemia, hemoglobinopathies

CABOT RINGS

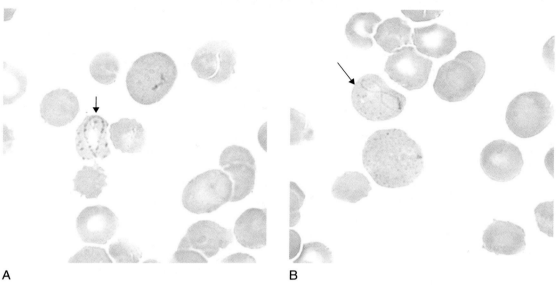

A

FIGURE 12–4A Cabot ring.

B

FIGURE 12–4B Cabot ring: figure eight.

COLOR: Dark blue to purple

SHAPE: Loop, ring, or figure eight; may look like beads on a string

NUMBER PER CELL: 1 to 2

COMPOSITION: Thought to be remnants of mitotic spindle

ASSOCIATED WITH: Myelodysplastic syndrome, megaloblastic anemia

> **NOTE:** This is a rare finding. May be confused with malaria (see Figure 21-1).

INCLUSIONS WITH SUPRAVITAL STAIN
Stained with New Methylene Blue

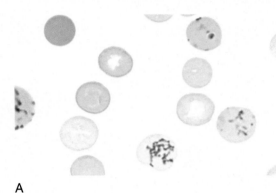

A

FIGURE 12–5A Reticulocytes.

CELL: Anuclear immature erythrocyte

COMPOSITION: Precipitated RNA

NUMBER: Two or more per cell

COLOR: Dark blue

ASSOCIATED WITH: Erythrocyte maturation

> **NOTE:** Supravital stains are taken up by living cells.

B

FIGURE 12–5B Heinz bodies.

CELL: Mature erythrocyte

COMPOSITION: Denatured hemoglobin

NUMBER: Single or multiple, generally membrane-bound

COLOR: Dark blue to purple

ASSOCIATED WITH: Unstable hemoglobin, some hemoglobinopathies, some erythrocyte enzyme deficiencies (e.g., glucose-6-phosphate dehydrogenase)

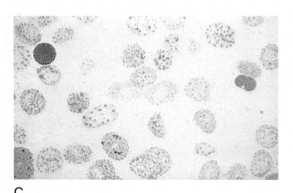

C

FIGURE 12–5C Hemoglobin H. (From the American Society for Hematology slide bank.)

CELL: Mature erythrocyte

COMPOSITION: Hemoglobin β chain tetramers

NUMBER: Multiple evenly dispersed inclusions described as "golf balls" or "raspberries"

COLOR: Dark blue

TABLE 12–1

Staining Qualities of Erythrocyte Inclusion Bodies

Inclusion	Composition	Wright-Giemsa stain	Appearance in Wright-Giemsa stain	New Methylene Blue (or other Supravital stain)	Appearance in New Methylene Blue stain	Prussian Blue (Iron)	Appearance in Prussian Blue iron stain
Howell-Jolly body	DNA	+		+	NA	0	NA
Basophilic stippling	RNA	+		+	NA	0	NA
Pappenheimer body	Iron	+		+	NA	+	
Cabot ring	Remnant of mitotic spindle	+		+	NA	0	NA
Reticulocyte	RNA	NA	NA	+		0	NA
Heinz body	Unstable hemoglobin	0	NA	+		0	NA
Hemoglobin H	β chain tetramers	0	NA	+		0	NA

+, Positive; 0, negative. *DNA*, Deoxyribonucleic acid; *NA*, not applicable; *RNA*, ribonucleic acid.

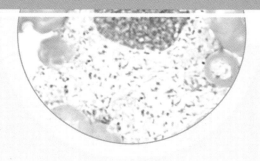

CHAPTER 13

DISEASES AFFECTING ERYTHROCYTES

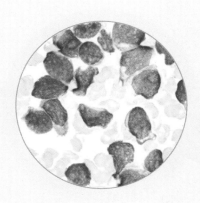

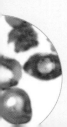

MICROCYTIC HYPOCHROMIC
IRON DEFICIENCY ANEMIA

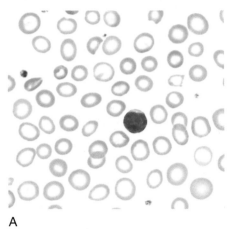

A

FIGURE 13–1A Severe iron deficiency anemia (peripheral blood [PB] ×500).

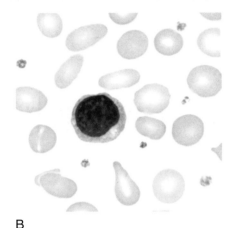

B

FIGURE 13–1B Iron deficiency anemia (PB ×1000).

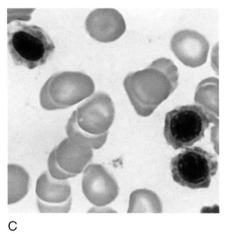

C

FIGURE 13–1C Iron deficiency anemia (bone marrow [BM] ×1000; showing shaggy cytoplasm).

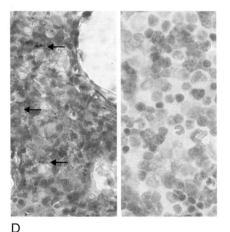

D

FIGURE 13–1D Prussian blue dye on bone marrow aspirate smears (500 ×). Normal iron stores (left). Absence of iron stores (right).
(From Keohane E.A., Smith L., Walenga J. (Eds.) (2016). Rodak's hematology: clinical principles and applications. (5th ed.). St. Louis: Saunders Elsevier.)

Peripheral Blood: Erythrocytes are hypochromic and microcytic; large variation in size; possible thrombocytosis

---

Although characteristic findings for disease states are listed, not all may be present in one patient. The most common ones are depicted.

β-THALASSEMIA MINOR
Genotypes: β/β^+ β/β^0 $\beta/\delta\beta^0$ $\beta/\delta\beta^{Lepore}$

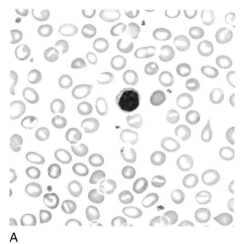

A

FIGURE 13–2A β-Thalassemia minor (PB ×500).

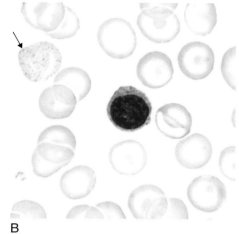

B

FIGURE 13–2B β-Thalassemia minor (PB ×1000).

Peripheral Blood: Microcytosis, slight hypochromia, target cells, basophilic stippling

NOTE: The presence of basophilic stippling (*arrow*) is common in thalassemia minor but not in iron deficiency anemia.

β-THALASSEMIA MAJOR
Genotypes: β^0/β^0 β^+/β^+ β^0/β^+ $\delta\beta^{Lepore}/\delta\beta^{Lepore}$

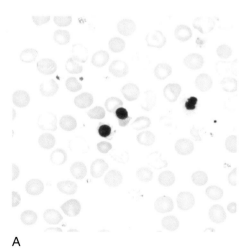

A

FIGURE 13–3A β-Thalassemia major (PB ×500).

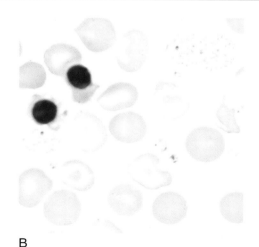

B

FIGURE 13–3B β-Thalassemia major (PB ×1000).

Peripheral Blood: Marked variation in size and shape, numerous nucleated erythrocytes, microcytes, hypochromia, target cells, basophilic stippling, teardrop cells, schistocytes, polychromasia

α-THALASSEMIA MINOR
Genotypes: $--/\alpha\alpha$, $-\alpha/-\alpha$, Hemoglobin H $--/-\alpha$

Peripheral Blood: Microcytes, hypochromia, marked poikilocytosis, target cells, polychromasia. α-Thalassemia minor ($--/\alpha\alpha$, $-\alpha/-\alpha$) has red cell morphology similar to β-thalassemia and as such is not represented here (see Figure 13–2, A and B, 12–5, C)

α-THALASSEMIA MAJOR
Hemoglobin Bart Hydrops Fetalis Syndrome
Genotype: $--/--$ (γ_4)

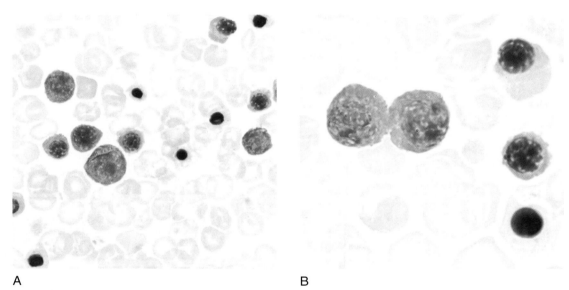

A

B

FIGURE 13–4A Bart hemoglobin (PB ×500).

FIGURE 13–4B Bart hemoglobin (PB ×1000).

Peripheral Blood: Numerous nucleated erythrocytes, marked variation in size, hypochromia, variable polychromasia, macrocytes

MACROCYTIC NORMOCHROMIC
NONMEGALOBLASTIC ANEMIA

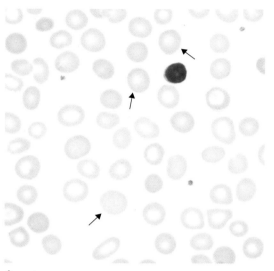

A

FIGURE 13–5A Macrocytic (nonmegaloblastic) (PB ×500).

B

FIGURE 13–5B Macrocytic (nonmegaloblastic) (PB ×1000).

Peripheral Blood: Round macrocytes, leukocyte and platelet counts usually normal

Bone Marrow: No megaloblastic changes

ASSOCIATED WITH: Normal newborn, liver disease, chronic alcoholism

MEGALOBLASTIC ANEMIA

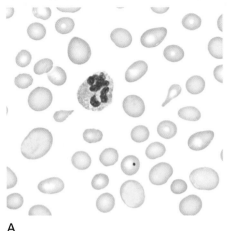

A

FIGURE 13–6A Megaloblastic anemia (PB ×500).

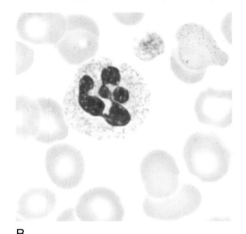

B

FIGURE 13–6B Megaloblastic anemia (PB ×1000).

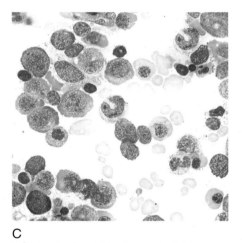

C

FIGURE 13–6C Megaloblastic anemia (BM original ×500).

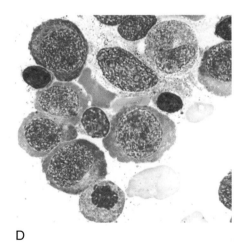

D

FIGURE 13–6D Megaloblastic anemia (BM original ×1000).

Peripheral Blood: Pancytopenia, hypersegmentation of neutrophils, oval macrocytes, teardrop cells, Howell-Jolly bodies, nucleated erythrocytes, basophilic stippling, schistocytes, spherocytes, target cells, giant platelets

NOTE: Characteristic triad of abnormalities: pancytopenia, oval macrocytes, and hypersegmented neutrophils

Bone Marrow: Hypercellular, asynchrony (trilineage) with nuclear maturation lagging behind cytoplasmic maturation, giant bands, giant metamyelocytes, hypersegmented neutrophils

ASSOCIATED WITH: Vitamin B_{12} deficiency, folate deficiency, myelodysplastic syndrome

NORMOCYTIC NORMOCHROMIC
APLASTIC ANEMIA

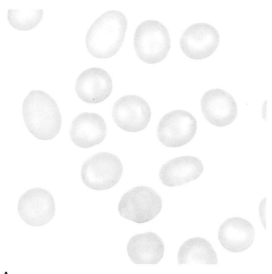

A

FIGURE 13–7A Aplastic anemia (PB ×1000).

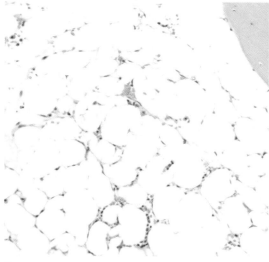

B

FIGURE 13–7B Aplastic anemia (BM biopsy ×1000).

Peripheral Blood: Pancytopenia, normocytic, normochromic (occasional macrocytes)

Bone Marrow: Hypocellular; lymphocytes may predominate

ASSOCIATED WITH: Bone marrow failure

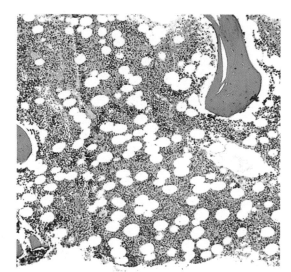

C

FIGURE 13–7C Representative core biopsy section showing normal cellularity, approximately 50% fat and 50% hematopoietic cells (hematoxylin and eosin, 50×). (From Keohane E.A., Smith L., Walenga J. (Eds.) (2016). Rodak's hematology: clinical principles and applications. (5th ed.). St. Louis: Saunders Elsevier.)

IMMUNE HEMOLYTIC ANEMIA

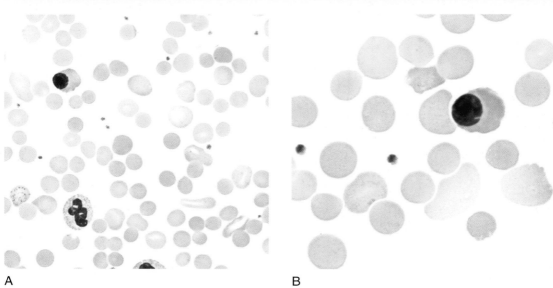

A

FIGURE 13–8A Immune hemolytic anemia (PB ×500).

B

FIGURE 13–8B Immune hemolytic anemia (PB ×1000).

Peripheral Blood: Spherocytes, schistocytes, polychromasia, nucleated erythrocytes

ASSOCIATED WITH: Autoimmune, alloimmune anemia (see also hemolytic disease of the fetus and newborn, Figure 13–9), drug-induced hemolytic anemia

NOTE: Erythrocyte morphology varies with cause and severity of disease.

HEMOLYTIC DISEASE OF THE FETUS AND NEWBORN

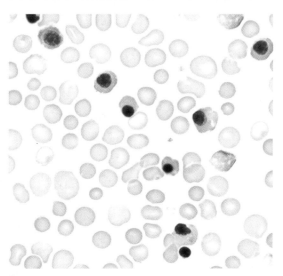

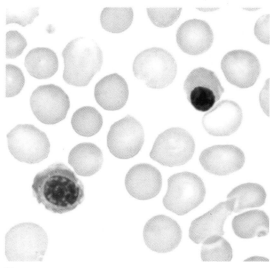

A

FIGURE 13–9A Hemolytic disease of the fetus and newborn (PB ×500).

B

FIGURE 13–9B Hemolytic disease of the fetus and newborn (PB ×1000).

Peripheral Blood: Polychromasia, increased number of nucleated erythrocytes, macrocytic/normochromic, spherocytes (more common in ABO incompatibility)

ASSOCIATED WITH: Fetal-maternal Rh and/or ABO incompatibility

NOTE: Normal newborns have some nucleated erythrocytes (see Chapter 23).

HEREDITARY SPHEROCYTOSIS

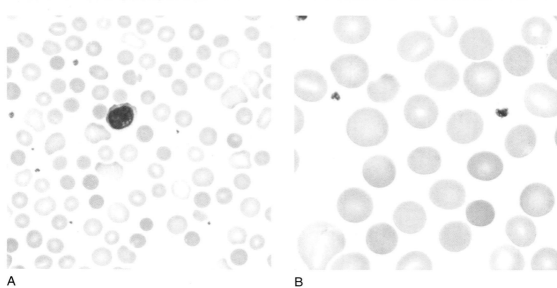

A

FIGURE 13–10A Hereditary spherocytosis (PB ×500).

B

FIGURE 13–10B Hereditary spherocytosis (PB ×1000).

Peripheral Blood: Spherocytes (variable in number), polychromasia; nucleated erythrocytes possible

ASSOCIATED WITH: Red cell membrane defects

HEREDITARY ELLIPTOCYTOSIS

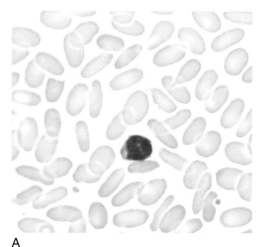

A

FIGURE 13–11A Hereditary elliptocytosis (PB ×500).

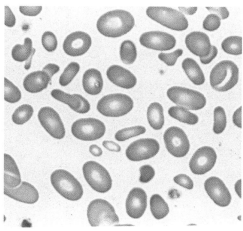

B

FIGURE 13–11B Hereditary pyropoikilocytosis: before incubation (PB ×500).

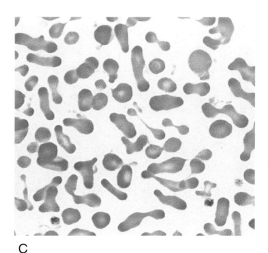

C

FIGURE 13–11C Hereditary pyropoikilocytosis: with incubation at 41° to 45° C for 1 hour (PB ×500).

Peripheral Blood: More than 25% elliptocytes, usually more than 60% elliptocytes; indices are normocytic, normochromic

ASSOCIATED WITH: Red cell membrane defects

VARIANTS OF ELLIPTOCYTOSIS

HEMOLYTIC
Peripheral Blood: Microelliptocytes, schistocytes, spherocytes (not depicted)

ASSOCIATED WITH: Red cell membrane defects

PYROPOIKILOCYTOSIS
Peripheral Blood: Elliptocytes, schistocytes, microspherocytes (see Figure 11–4, B)

ASSOCIATED WITH: Red cell membrane defects

MICROANGIOPATHIC HEMOLYTIC ANEMIA

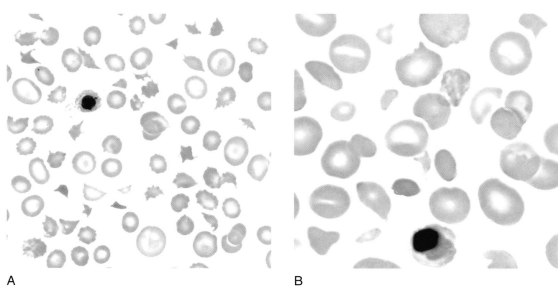

A

FIGURE 13–12A Microangiopathic hemolytic anemia (PB ×500).

B

FIGURE 13–12B Microangiopathic hemolytic anemia (PB ×1000).

Peripheral Blood: Schistocytes, spherocytes, polychromasia, nucleated erythrocytes, decreased platelet count

ASSOCIATED WITH: Thrombotic thrombocytopenic purpura, hemolytic uremic syndrome, HELLP syndrome (Hemolytic anemia, Elevated Liver enzymes and Low Platelet count), disseminated intravascular coagulation, hypertensive crises

NOTE: The degree of morphological change correlates directly with the severity of the disease.

HEMOGLOBIN CC DISEASE

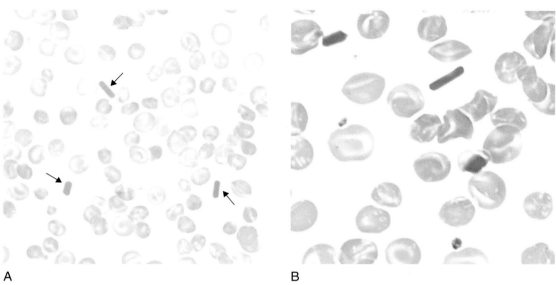

A

FIGURE 13–13A Hemoglobin CC (PB ×500).

B

FIGURE 13–13B Hemoglobin CC (PB ×1000).

Peripheral Blood: Polychromasia, target cells, spherocytes, microcytes, intracellular and/or extracellular rod-shaped crystals possible

ASSOCIATED WITH: Homozygous hemoglobin C (see Figure 11–7)

HEMOGLOBIN SS DISEASE

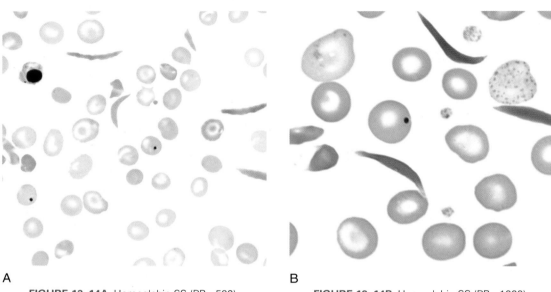

A

FIGURE 13–14A Hemoglobin SS (PB ×500).

B

FIGURE 13–14B Hemoglobin SS (PB ×1000).

Peripheral Blood: Sickle cells (in crises), target cells, nucleated erythrocytes, schistocytes, Howell-Jolly bodies, basophilic stippling, Pappenheimer bodies, polychromasia, increased leukocyte count with neutrophilia, thrombocytosis

ASSOCIATED WITH: Homozygous hemoglobin S (see Figure 11–6)

HEMOGLOBIN SC DISEASE

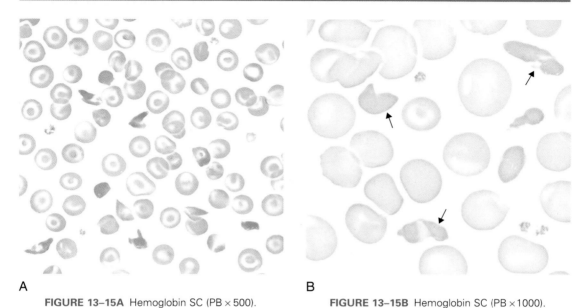

A

FIGURE 13–15A Hemoglobin SC (PB × 500).

B

FIGURE 13–15B Hemoglobin SC (PB × 1000).

Peripheral Blood: Few sickle cells, target cells, intraerythrocytic crystals; crystalline aggregates of hemoglobin SC may protrude from the erythrocyte membrane

ASSOCIATED WITH: Hemoglobin SC (see Figure 11–8)

CHAPTER 14

NUCLEAR AND CYTOPLASMIC CHANGES IN LEUKOCYTES

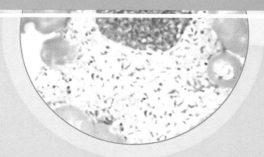

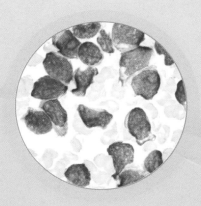

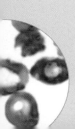

HYPOSEGMENTATION OF NEUTROPHILS

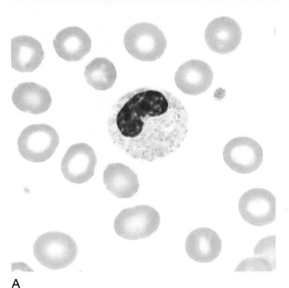

A

FIGURE 14–1A Hyposegmentation: peanut-shaped nucleus.

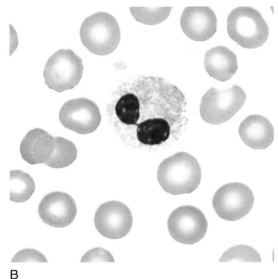

B

FIGURE 14–1B Hyposegmentation: bilobed nucleus.

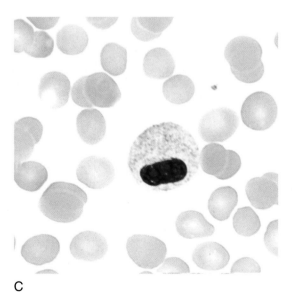

C

FIGURE 14–1C Non-segmented nucleus.

DESCRIPTION: Peanut-shaped, bilobed or non-segmented, granulocyte nucleus with the coarse chromatin of a mature cell

ASSOCIATED WITH: Pelger-Hüet anomaly, pseudo-Pelger-Hüet anomaly

NOTE: Pelger-Hüet anomaly is inherited and affects the majority of granulocytes. Pseudo-Pelger-Hüet is acquired, affects less than 50% of granulocytes, and is usually accompanied by other morphologic indications of malignancy, such as those seen in myeloproliferative or myelodysplastic disorders (see Chapters 17 and 18).

All photomicrographs are ×1000 with Wright–Giemsa stain unless stated otherwise.

HYPERSEGMENTATION OF NEUTROPHILS

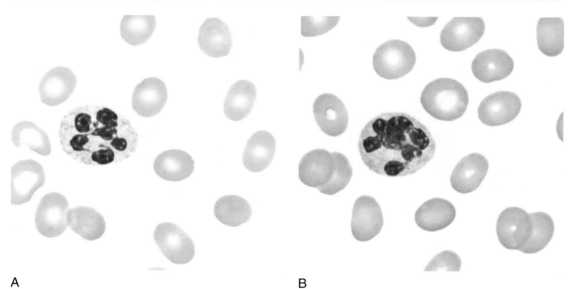

A

FIGURE 14–2A Hypersegmented neutrophil.

B

FIGURE 14–2B Hypersegmented neutrophil.

DESCRIPTION: Six or more lobes in granulocyte nucleus

ASSOCIATED WITH: Megaloblastic anemias, chronic infections, myelodysplastic syndrome, rarely inherited

VACUOLATION IN NEUTROPHILS

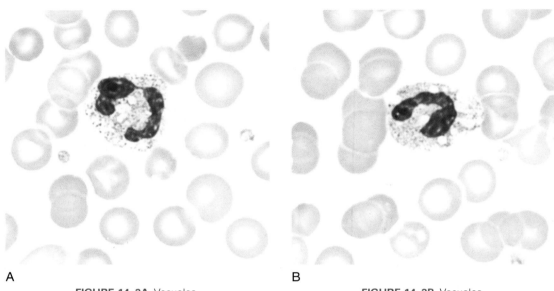

A

FIGURE 14–3A Vacuoles.

B

FIGURE 14–3B Vacuoles.

DESCRIPTION: Unstained circular area within the cytoplasm

NUMBER: Few to many

ASSOCIATED WITH: Bacterial or fungal infection, poisoning, burns, chemotherapy, artifact

> **NOTE:** Vacuoles rarely may contain microorganisms or pigment. Vacuoles are seen in normal monocytes and do not suggest infection.

DÖHLE BODY

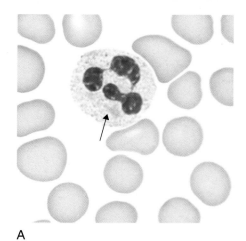

A

FIGURE 14–4A Döhle body.

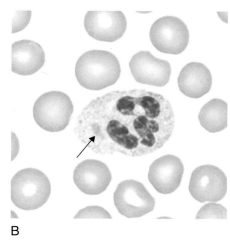

B

FIGURE 14–4B Döhle body.

DESCRIPTION: Gray-blue, variably shaped inclusion in cytoplasm

COMPOSITION: Ribosomal RNA

NUMBER: Single or multiple

ASSOCIATED WITH: Wide range of conditions, including bacterial infection, sepsis, and normal pregnancy

> **NOTE:** May be seen in cells with toxic granulation or on same slide with toxic granulation.
> (See Figure 14–5, B.)

TOXIC GRANULATION

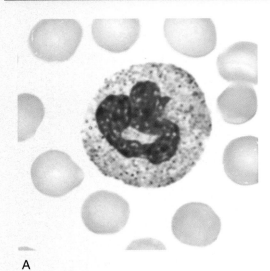

A

FIGURE 14–5A Toxic granulation.

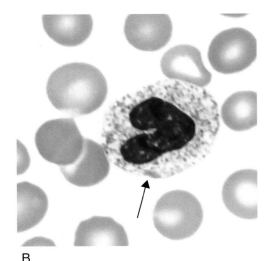

B

FIGURE 14–5B Toxic granulation and Döhle body (*arrow*). Cytoplasm may retain blue color caused by cell's early release from bone marrow.

DESCRIPTION: Prominent dark purple-black granules in the cytoplasm of neutrophils, unevenly distributed

COMPOSITION: Primary granules

NUMBER: Few to many

ASSOCIATED WITH: Wide range of conditions including bacterial infection and sepsis and following administration of granulocyte colony-stimulating factor

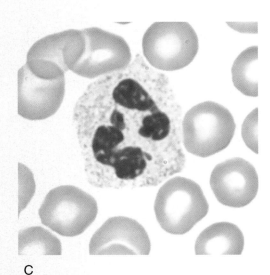

C

FIGURE 14–5C Normal segmented neutrophil for comparison.

HYPOGRANULATION/AGRANULATION IN NEUTROPHILS

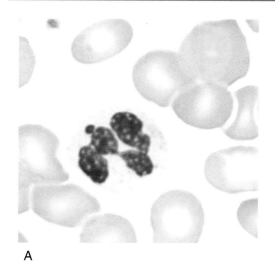

A

FIGURE 14–6A Hypogranulation.

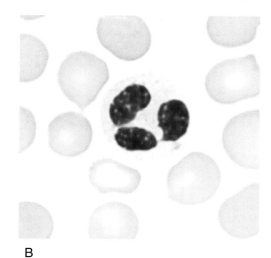

B

FIGURE 14–6B Agranulation.

DESCRIPTION: Decreased number or absence of specific granules giving the cytoplasm a colorless appearance

ASSOCIATED WITH: Myelodysplastic syndrome, myeloproliferative neoplasms, infection

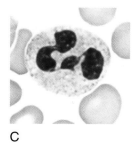

C

FIGURE 14–6C Normal segmented neutrophil for comparison.

REACTIVE LYMPHOCYTES

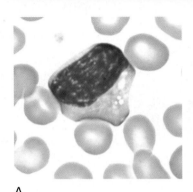

A

FIGURE 14–7A Reactive lymphocyte, vacuolated cytoplasm.

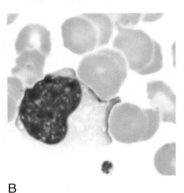

B

FIGURE 14–7B Reactive lymphocyte, peripheral basophilia.

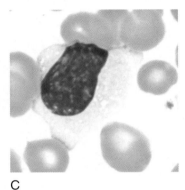

C

FIGURE 14–7C Reactive lymphocyte, cytoplasm indented by adjacent cells.

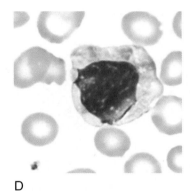

D

FIGURE 14–7D Reactive lymphocyte, radial basophilia.

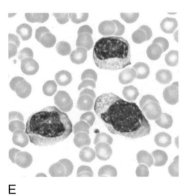

E

FIGURE 14–7E Reactive lymphocytes, characteristic of viral diseases, such as infectious mononucleosis (PB ×500).

DESCRIPTION: 10 to 30 μm; Pleomorphic; easily indented by surrounding cells

NUCLEUS: Irregular
Nucleoli: Occasionally present
Chromatin: When compared with that of a resting lymphocyte, chromatin is coarse to fine and dispersed

CYTOPLASM: Pale blue to deeply basophilic, may stain unevenly with peripheral or radial basophilia
Granules: May have increased numbers of azurophilic granules
Vacuoles: Occasional

ASSOCIATED WITH: Viral infections and other antigenic stimulation, including organ transplantation

Refer to Appendix Table A-2 for a comparison of monocytes and reactive lymphocytes.

CHAPTER 15

ACUTE MYELOID LEUKEMIA

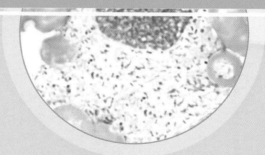

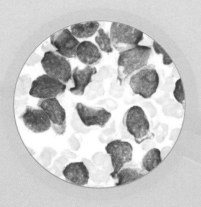

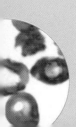

The World Health Organization (WHO) *Classification of Tumours and Haematopoietic and Lymphoid Tissues* is based on morphology; immunophenotyping; genetic features, including karyotype and molecular testing; and clinical features. WHO lists the characteristic features of acute myeloid leukemia (AML) as increased bone marrow cellularity with 20% or more blasts, variable white blood cell count, anemia, and thrombocytopenia in the peripheral blood.

AML is separated into four categories:

1. Acute myeloid leukemia with recurrent genetic abnormalities.
2. Acute myeloid leukemia with myelodysplasia-related changes.*
3. Therapy-related myeloid neoplasms.*
4. Acute myeloid leukemia, not otherwise specified.

This atlas presents characteristic peripheral blood and bone marrow morphology for each of the AMLs with recurrent genetic abnormalities and those not otherwise specified, together with the associated cytochemical reactions, genetic abnormalities, and immunophenotypes.

*Diagnosis is, in part, based on patient presentation and as such will not be addressed in this atlas.

ACUTE MYELOID LEUKEMIA, MINIMALLY DIFFERENTIATED
FAB† M0

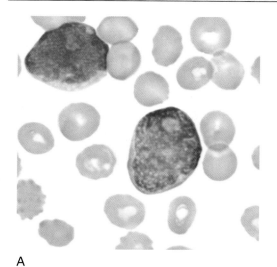

A

FIGURE 15–1A Peripheral blood (×1000).

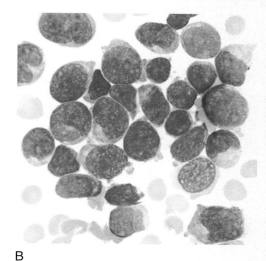

B

FIGURE 15–1B Bone marrow (×500).

MORPHOLOGY:
Peripheral Blood: Large agranular blasts
Bone Marrow: Large agranular blasts

CYTOCHEMISTRY:
Myeloperoxidase: Negative
Sudan Black B: Negative
Nonspecific Esterase: Negative

GENETICS:
Recurrent genetic abnormalities: not defined.

IMMUNOPHENOTYPE:
CD13⁺, CD33⁺, CD117⁺, HLA-DR±, CD34±, CD38⁺

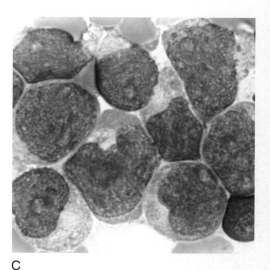

C

FIGURE 15–1C Bone marrow (×1000).

†French-American-British classification of acute leukemia.

ACUTE MYELOID LEUKEMIA WITHOUT MATURATION
FAB M1

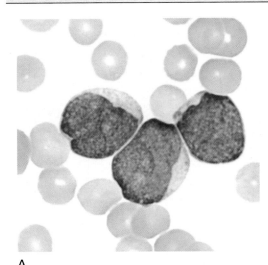

A

FIGURE 15–2A Peripheral blood (×1000).

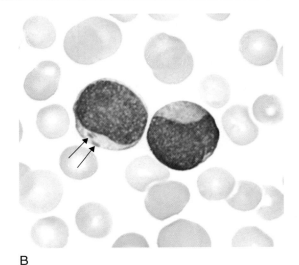

B

FIGURE 15–2B Peripheral blood: Auer rods in myeloblast (×1000). Auer rods are composed of fused primary granules, usually rod shaped but may be round in appearance. Single or multiple Auer rods may be seen in malignant myeloblasts and malignant promyelocytes.

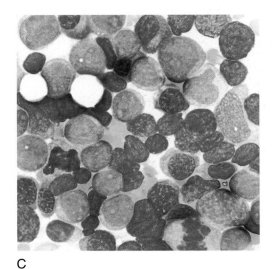

C

FIGURE 15–2C Bone marrow (×500).

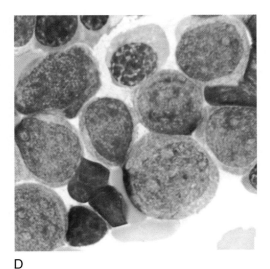

D

FIGURE 15–2D Bone marrow (×1000).

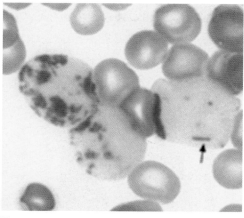

E

FIGURE 15–2E Positive myeloperoxidase stain.

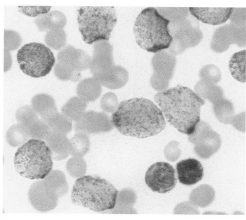

F

FIGURE 15–2F Positive Sudan Black B stain.

MORPHOLOGY:
Peripheral Blood: Blasts ± Auer rods (see Figure 15–2, A and B)
Bone Marrow: 90% or higher of nonerythroid cells are blasts

CYTOCHEMISTRY:
Myeloperoxidase: Positive (see Figure 15–2, E)
Sudan Black B: Positive (see Figure 15–2, F)
Nonspecific Esterase: Negative

GENETICS:
Recurrent genetic abnormalities: not defined.

IMMUNOPHENOTYPE:
CD13$^+$, CD33$^+$, CD34$^\pm$, HLA-DR$^\pm$, CD117$^+$

ACUTE MYELOID LEUKEMIA WITH MATURATION
FAB M2

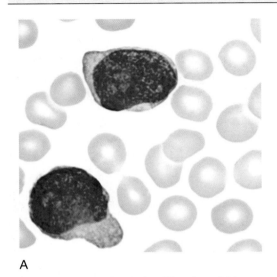

A

FIGURE 15–3A Peripheral blood Type I myeloblast (×1000).

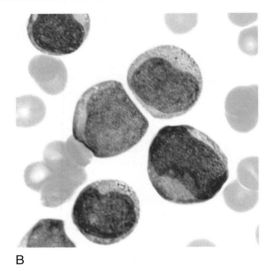

B

FIGURE 15–3B Peripheral blood Type II myeloblast (×1000).

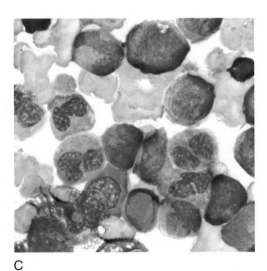

C

FIGURE 15–3C Bone marrow (×500).

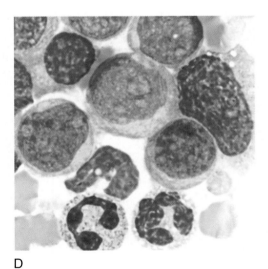

D

FIGURE 15–3D Bone marrow (×1000).

MORPHOLOGY:

Peripheral Blood: Blasts with some maturation $\pm$ Auer rods (see Figures 15–2, A and B)
Bone Marrow: Blasts, some with large azurophilic granules, perinuclear hof $\pm$ Auer rods
Less than 90% of nonerythroid cells are blasts
10% or higher neutrophilic component
Less than 20% monocytic component

CYTOCHEMISTRY:

Myeloperoxidase: Positive (see Figure 15–2, E)
Sudan Black B: Positive (see Figure 15–2, F)

GENETICS:

Subset with t(8;21) is designated as AML with recurrent genetic abnormalities. In this subset, blasts are large with abundant basophilic cytoplasm, azurophilic granules, and possible perinuclear hofs.

IMMUNOPHENOTYPE:

CD13$^+$, CD33$^+$, CD65$^+$, CD11b$^+$, CD15$^+$, HLA-DR$^\pm$

ACUTE PROMYELOCYTIC LEUKEMIA

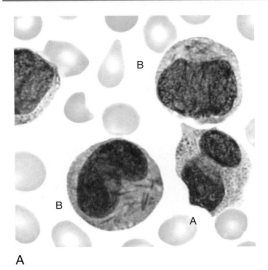

A

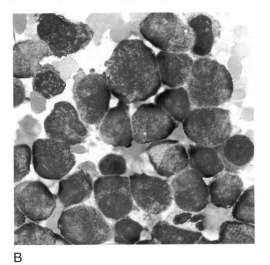

B

FIGURE 15–4A Peripheral blood. A, Hypergranular promyelocyte (×1000); B, Faggot cells.

FIGURE 15–4B Bone marrow (×500).

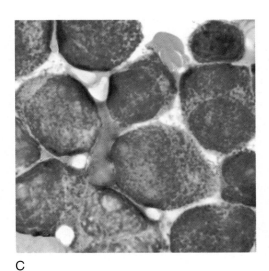

C

FIGURE 15–4C Bone marrow (×1000).

MORPHOLOGY:

Peripheral Blood: White blood cell count may be low or only slightly elevated

Blasts, hypergranular promyelocytes, cytoplasm gray to blue, nucleus may be folded or bilobed

Multiple Auer rods possible, may be in bundles (Faggot cells), schistocytes

Bone Marrow: Blasts, hypergranular promyelocytes, nuclei often bilobed or kidney shaped

± Multiple Auer rods

CYTOCHEMISTRY:

Myeloperoxidase: Strongly positive (see Figure 15–2, E)

Sudan Black B: Strongly positive (see Figure 15–2, F)

GENETICS:

t(15;17) is sufficient for diagnosis as AML with recurrent genetic abnormalities regardless of blast/promyelocyte count.[‡]

IMMUNOPHENOTYPE:

$CD13^{\pm}$, $CD33^{+}$, $CD34^{-}$, HLA-DR^{-}

NOTE: Acute promyelocytic leukemia may be associated with disseminated intravascular coagulopathy.

[‡]1. Abnormal promyelocytes are considered blast equivalents for the purpose of diagnosis.

ACUTE PROMYELOCYTIC LEUKEMIA: MICROGRANULAR VARIANT

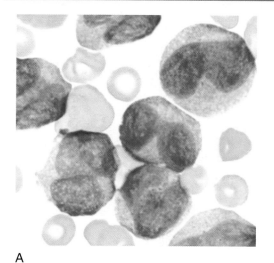

A

FIGURE 15–5A Peripheral blood (×1000).

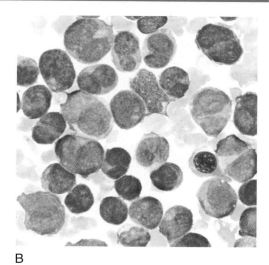

B

FIGURE 15–5B Bone marrow (×500).

MORPHOLOGY:
Peripheral Blood: White blood cell count markedly elevated, deeply notched nuclei
Cytoplasm may appear agranular because of small size of granules, which are evident with electron microscopy
Bone Marrow: Agranular promyelocytes, with deeply notched nuclei

CYTOCHEMISTRY:
Myeloperoxidase: Strongly positive (see Figure 15–2, E)
Sudan Black B: Strongly positive (see Figure 15–2, F)

GENETICS:
t(15;17) is sufficient for diagnosis as AML with recurrent genetic abnormalities regardless of blast/promyelocyte count.

IMMUNOPHENOTYPE:
CD13$^\pm$, CD33$^+$, CD34$^-$, HLA-DR$^-$, CD64$^+$, CD117$^\pm$

NOTE: Microgranular promyelocytes can be confused morphologically with monocyte precursors.

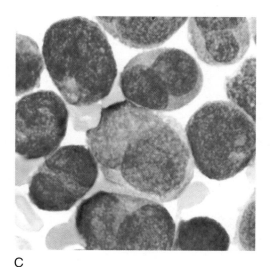

C

FIGURE 15–5C Bone marrow (×1000).

ACUTE MYELOMONOCYTIC LEUKEMIA
FAB M4

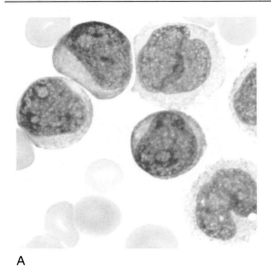

A

FIGURE 15–6A Peripheral blood (×1000).

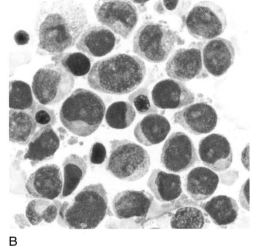

B

FIGURE 15–6B Bone marrow (×500).

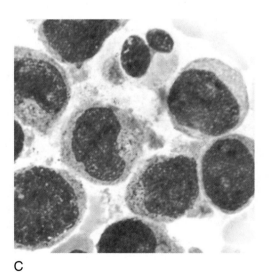

C

FIGURE 15–6C Bone marrow (×1000).

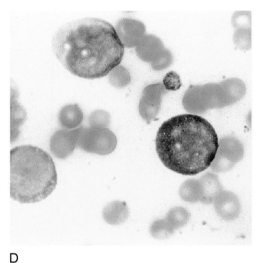

D

FIGURE 15–6D Positive naphthol-AS-D chloroacetate esterase (specific) stain.

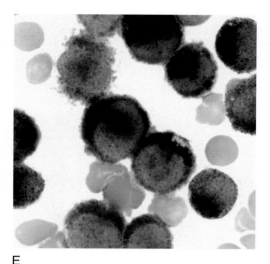

E

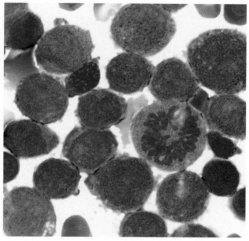

F

FIGURE 15–6E Positive α-naphthyl acetate esterase (nonspecific) esterase stain in monocytes.

FIGURE 15–6F α-Naphthyl acetate esterase stain inhibited by NaFl.

MORPHOLOGY:

Peripheral Blood: Myeloblasts, promyelocytes, and other immature myeloid precursors

Monoblasts, promonocytes, and monocytes; frequently more mature than those seen in bone marrow

± Auer rods (see Figure 15–2, B)

Bone Marrow: Monoblasts are large with abundant, moderate basophilic cytoplasm; some with folded nuclei, one or more prominent nucleoli

Promonocytes have irregular, convoluted nucleus, cytoplasm slightly basophilic; granules; occasional vacuoles

± Auer rods

Granulocytes and their precursors and monocytes and their precursors each comprise 20% or higher

CYTOCHEMISTRY:

Myeloperoxidase: Positive (see Figure 15–2, E)

Specific Esterase: Naphthol-AS-D chloroacetate esterase is positive in granulocytic cells and weak in monocytic cells (see Figure 15–6, D)

Nonspecific Esterase:

- α-Naphthyl acetate esterase: positive in monocytic cells (Figure 15–6, E); inhibited by NaFl (Figure 15–6, F)
- α-Naphthyl butyrate esterase: positive in monocytic cells (see Figure 15–8, D)

GENETICS:

Recurrent genetic abnormalities: not defined.

NOTE: inv(16) or t(16;16) and abnormal eosinophils are excluded from this category.

IMMUNOPHENOTYPE:

CD13+, CD33+, CD14+, CD4+, CD11b+, CD64+, CD15+, CD36+

ACUTE MYELOID LEUKEMIA WITH inv(16) (13.1;q22) OR t(16;16) (p13.1;q22); CBFB-MYH11

Acute Myeloid Leukemia with Abnormal Marrow Eosinophils

FAB M4EO

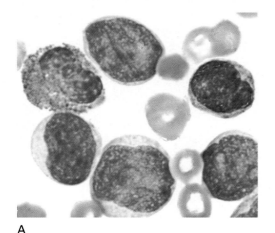

A

FIGURE 15–7A Peripheral blood (×1000).

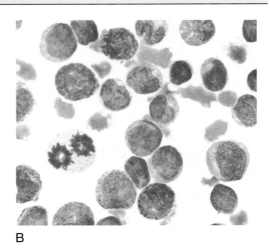

B

FIGURE 15–7B Bone marrow (×500).

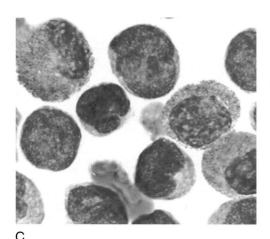

C

FIGURE 15–7C Bone marrow (×1000).

MORPHOLOGY:

Peripheral Blood: Myeloblasts, promyelocytes, and other immature myeloid precursors
Monoblasts, promonocytes, and monocytes
± Auer rods (see Figure 15–2, B)

Bone Marrow: Monoblasts are large with abundant moderate basophilic cytoplasm; some with folded nuclei,
one or more prominent nucleoli
Promonocytes have irregular, convoluted nucleus, cytoplasm slightly basophilic; granules; occasional vacuoles
Eosinophils increased and dysplastic with many large granules, some basophilic
± Auer rods

CYTOCHEMISTRY:

Myeloperoxidase: Positive (see Figure 15–2, E)
Nonspecific Esterase: Positive (see Figure 15–6, E)
Specific Esterase: Weakly positive in abnormal eosinophils

GENETICS:

Recurrent genetic abnormality: inv(16) (p13.1;q22) or t(16;16)(p13.1;q22); CBFB-MYH11

NOTE: These genetic abnormalities are diagnostic of AML and do not require a 20% or higher blast count.

IMMUNOPHENOTYPE:

$CD34^+$, $CD117^+$, $CD13^+$, $CD33^+$, $CD15^+$, $CD4^+$, $CD11b^+$, $CD11c^+$, $CD14^+$, $CD64^+$, $CD36^+$, $CD65^+$

ACUTE MONOBLASTIC AND MONOCYTIC LEUKEMIA
FAB M5

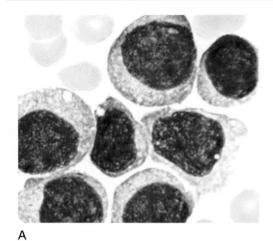

A

FIGURE 15–8A Peripheral blood: monoblasts predominate (×1000).

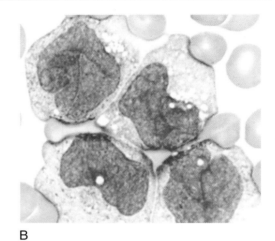

B

FIGURE 15–8B Peripheral blood: promonocytes predominate (×1000).

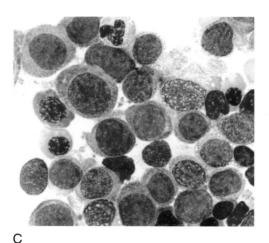

C

FIGURE 15–8C Bone marrow showing monoblast predominance (×500).

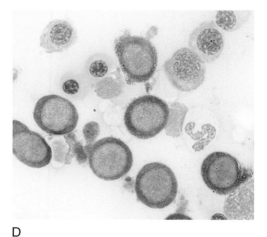

D

FIGURE 15–8D Positive α-naphthyl butyrate esterase (nonspecific) esterase stain.

MORPHOLOGY:

Peripheral Blood: Monoblasts, promonocytes

Bone Marrow: Monoblasts are large with abundant moderate basophilic cytoplasm, some with folded nuclei, one or more prominent nucleoli

Promonocytes have irregular, convoluted nucleus, cytoplasm slightly basophilic; granules; occasional vacuoles

80% or more have monocytic morphology

Granulocytic component less than 20%

NOTE: Monoblastic leukemia is diagnosed when 80% or more leukemic cells are monoblasts. In monocytic leukemia predominant cell type is promonocyte.

CYTOCHEMISTRY:

Myeloperoxidase: Negative

Nonspecific Esterase: Positive (see Figures 15–6, E, and 15–8, D)

GENETICS:

Subset with t(9;11)(p22;q23); MLLT3-MLL is diagnosed as AML with recurrent genetic abnormalities.

IMMUNOPHENOTYPE:

$CD33^+$, $CD13^+$, $CD4^+$, $CD14^+$, $CD11b^+$, $CD64^+$, $CD15^+$, $CD65^+$, $CD11c^+$, $CD36^+$, $CD68^+$, HLA-DR$^+$

ACUTE ERYTHROID LEUKEMIA
FAB M6a
(Erythroid/Myeloid Leukemia)

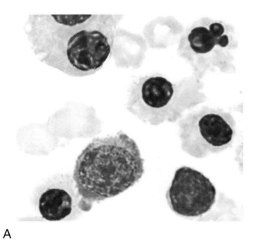

A

FIGURE 15–9A Peripheral blood (×1000).

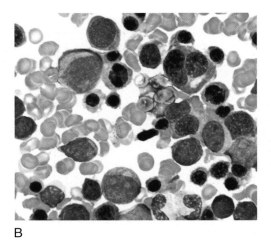

B

FIGURE 15–9B Bone marrow: erythroid/myeloid leukemia (×500).

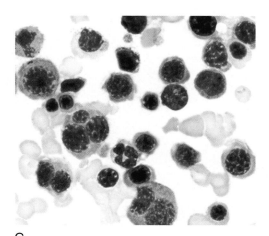

C

FIGURE 15–9C Bone marrow: pure erythroid leukemia (×500).

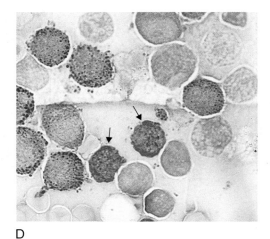

D

FIGURE 15–9D Positive periodic acid–Schiff stain.

MORPHOLOGY:
Peripheral Blood: Myeloblasts, ± Auer rods
Oval macrocytes, microcytes, dimorphic red blood cell population, ± basophilic stippling, dysplastic nucleated
  red blood cells, multiple nuclei, ± abnormal nuclear shapes (see Figure 18–1, A–D)
Bone Marrow: 20% or more of nonerythroid cells are myeloblasts, ± Auer rods
50% or more of all nucleated cells are erythroid precursors
Dysplastic erythroid precursors with megaloblastoid nuclei, round nuclei, fine chromatin, multiple nucleoli,
  nuclear bridging
Cytoplasm deeply basophilic, often contains vacuoles that may fuse together (see dyserythropoiesis, Figure 18–1,
  E–H)
Neutrophils: ± dysplastic changes
Megakaryocytes: ± dysplastic changes

CYTOCHEMISTRY:
Myeloperoxidase: Positive in myeloblasts (see Figure 15–2, E)
Sudan Black B: Positive in myeloblasts (see Figure 15–2, F)
Periodic Acid–Schiff: Positive in erythroblasts; either diffuse or block (see Figure 15–9, D)
Iron Stain: ± Ringed sideroblasts (see Figure 18–1, I)

GENETICS:
Recurrent genetic abnormalities: not defined.

IMMUNOPHENOTYPE:
Hemoglobin +, glycophorin +, $CD13^+$, $CD33^+$, $CD117^{\pm}$

FAB M6b
Pure Erythroid Leukemia

MORPHOLOGY:
Peripheral Blood: Dysplastic nucleated red blood cells, multiple nuclei, ± abnormal nuclear shapes
Oval macrocytes, microcytes, dimorphic red blood cell population, ± basophilic stippling

Bone Marrow: 80% or more erythroid precursors without evidence of a myeloid component
Immature erythroid cells with deeply basophilic cytoplasm, round nuclei, one or more nucleoli, vacuoles (some
  coalesced)

CYTOCHEMISTRY:
Myeloperoxidase: Negative
Sudan Black B: Negative
Nonspecific Esterase: Positive or negative
Periodic Acid–Schiff: Block positivity in erythroblasts (see Figure 15–9, D)
Iron Stain: ± Ringed sideroblasts (see Figure 18–1, I)

GENETICS:
Recurrent genetic abnormalities: not defined.

IMMUNOPHENOTYPE:
$CD71^+$, glycophorin +, hemoglobin +, $CD13^-$, $CD33^-$, $CD117^{\pm}$

ACUTE MEGAKARYOCYTIC LEUKEMIA
FAB M7

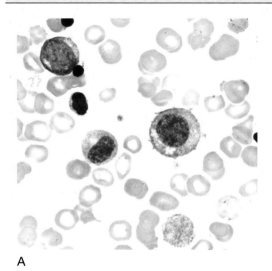

A

FIGURE 15–10A Peripheral blood (×500).

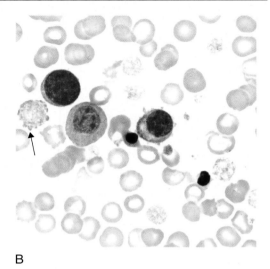

B

FIGURE 15–10B Peripheral blood (×500).

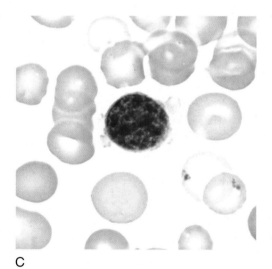

C

FIGURE 15–10C Micromegakaryocyte. Peripheral blood (×1000).

MORPHOLOGY:
Peripheral Blood: Blasts with budding cytoplasm
Micromegakaryocytes ± (see Figures 15–10, C, and 18–3, E)
Large atypical platelets with irregular borders (arrow)
Hypogranular neutrophils

Bone Marrow: Usually results in dry tap
20% or more blasts
50% or more of blasts are megakaryoblasts
Two types of blasts may be present:
SMALL BLASTS Resembling lymphoblasts, round nucleus, dense chromatin, scanty cytoplasm
LARGE BLASTS Fine nuclear chromatin, nucleoli, cytoplasm abundant, basophilic, agranular, ± pseudopods

CYTOCHEMISTRY:
Myeloperoxidase: Negative
Sudan Black B: Negative
Specific Esterase: Negative
Periodic Acid–Schiff: Positive or negative
Nonspecific Esterase: Focal positivity

GENETICS:
Recurrent genetic abnormalities: not defined.

NOTE: In infants may be associated with t(1:22)(p13;q13).

IMMUNOPHENOTYPE:
CD41+, CD61+, CD36+

CHAPTER 16

PRECURSOR LYMPHOID NEOPLASMS

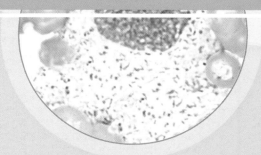

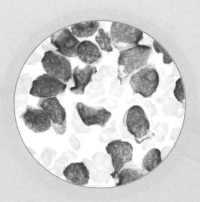

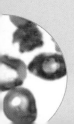

The World Health Organization classifies precursor lymphoid neoplasms into two major groups: B lymphoblastic leukemia/lymphoma and T lymphoblastic leukemia/lymphoma. Leukemia is primarily a disease of peripheral blood and bone marrow, whereas the primary site of involvement for lymphoma is the lymph system. Because this is an atlas of blood cells, only the leukemia morphology will be presented. Acute lymphoblastic leukemia (ALL) is not classified morphologically or by cytochemistry but by a combination of cytogenetic profiles, genotype, and immunophenotype. B lymphoblastic leukemia is subdivided into seven subtypes that are associated with recurrent genetic abnormalities (Box 16-1). Those cases of B-ALL that do not fall within one of these groups are classified as B lymphoblastic leukemia, not otherwise specified. Although 50% to 70% of patients with T-ALL do have abnormal karyotypes, none of the abnormalities is clearly associated with distinctive biologic features, and thus T-ALL is not further subdivided.

Lymphoblasts may be either small and homogeneous or large and heterogeneous. Further testing is needed to determine the phenotype and genotype.

BOX 16-1

B Lymphoblastic Leukemia/Lymphoma with Recurrent Genetic Abnormalities (2008 World Health Organization Classification)

B lymphoblastic leukemia/lymphoma with t(9;22)(q34;q11.2); *BCR-ABL1*
B lymphoblastic leukemia/lymphoma with t(v;11q23); *MLL* rearranged
B lymphoblastic leukemia/lymphoma with t(12;21)(p13;q22); *TEL-AML1(ETV6-RUNX1)*
B lymphoblastic leukemia/lymphoma with hyperdiploidy
B lymphoblastic leukemia/lymphoma with hypodiploidy
B lymphoblastic leukemia/lymphoma with t(5;14)(q31;q32); *IL3-IGH*
B lymphoblastic leukemia/lymphoma with t(1;19)(q23;p13.3); *E2A-PBX1 (TCF3-PBX1)*

From Swerdlow SH, Campo E, Harris NL, et al, (editors): *WHO classification of tumours of haematopoietic and lymphoid tissues*, ed 4, Lyon, France, IARC Press, 2008.

ACUTE LYMPHOBLASTIC LEUKEMIA, SMALL BLASTS

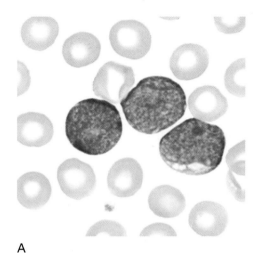

A

FIGURE 16–1A Peripheral blood (×1000).

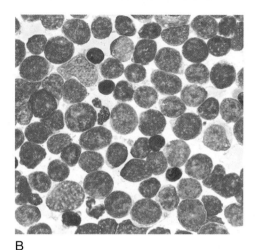

B

FIGURE 16–1B Bone marrow (×500).

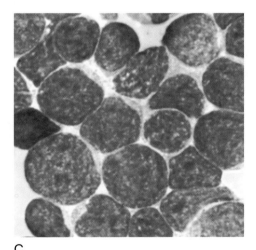

C

FIGURE 16–1C Bone marrow demonstrating homogeneous blasts in acute lymphoblastic leukemia (×1000).

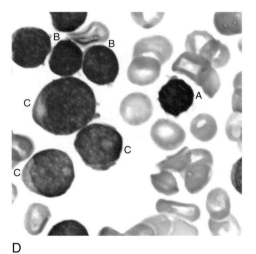

D

FIGURE 16–1D Bone marrow demonstrating the comparison between hematogones and lymphoblasts. A, Normal lymphocyte; B, hematogones; and C, lymphoblasts (×1000).

MORPHOLOGY:

Peripheral Blood: ± Blasts, small blasts (about one to two-and-a-half times the size of a resting lymphocyte) with scant blue cytoplasm, condensed chromatin and indistinct nucleoli, thrombocytopenia

Bone Marrow: 20% or more of all nucleated cells make up a homogeneous population of blasts

NOTE: Hematogones (immature B cells) may be seen in bone marrow and peripheral blood of newborns or in patients during bone marrow recovery. Care must be taken not to confuse hematogones with small lymphoblasts (see Figures 16–1, D and 23–4).

ACUTE LYMPHOBLASTIC LEUKEMIA, LARGE BLASTS

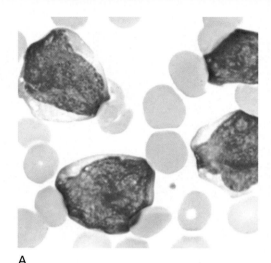

A

FIGURE 16–2A Peripheral blood (×1000).

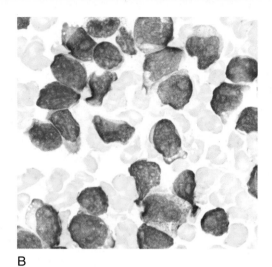

B

FIGURE 16–2B Bone marrow (×500).

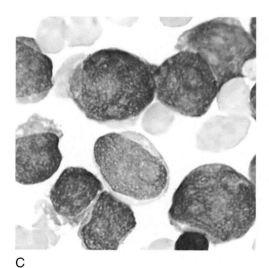

C

FIGURE 16–2C Bone marrow (×1000).

MORPHOLOGY:

Peripheral Blood: Blasts two to three times the size of a resting lymphocyte, moderate cytoplasm, irregular nuclear membrane, prominent nucleoli, thrombocytopenia, morphologically difficult to distinguish from acute myeloid leukemia

Bone Marrow: 20% or more of all nucleated cells comprise a heterogeneous population of blasts

CHAPTER 17

MYELOPROLIFERATIVE NEOPLASMS

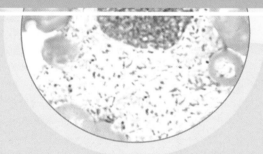

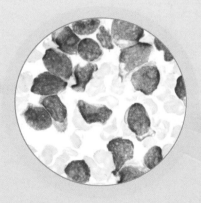

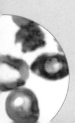

M yeloproliferative neoplasms (MPN) are clonal hematopoietic stem cell diseases with expansion, excessive production, and overaccumulation of erythrocytes, granulocytes, and platelets individually or in some combination.

The World Health Organization *Classification of Tumors of the Hematopoietic and Lymphoid Tissues* has divided these disorders into four major categories:

1. Chronic myelogenous leukemia, BCR–ABL1+ (CML)
2. Polycythemia vera (PV)
3. Essential thrombocythemia (ET)
4. Primary myelofibrosis (PMF)

These neoplasms have common clinical features, laboratory findings, and pathogenetic similarities (Table 17-1).

WHO identified several other rare myeloproliferative neoplasms that will not be covered in this atlas.

TABLE 17-1

Laboratory Features of Myeloproliferative Neoplasms				
Parameter	CML	PV	ET	PMF
WBC	Increased	Normal or increased	Normal or slightly increased	Normal, increased, or decreased
RBC	Normal or decreased	Increased	Normal or slightly decreased	Normal or decreased
Platelets	Normal or increased	Normal or increased	Increased	Normal, increased, or decreased
Molecular abnormalities	BCR-ABL1	JAK2 V617F or other JAK2 mutation	± JAK2	± JAK2

CML, Chronic myelogenous leukemia; *ET,* essential thrombocythemia; *JAK2,* Janus kinase 2; *PMF,* primary myelofibrosis; *PV,* polycythemia vera; *RBC,* red blood cells; *WBC,* white blood cells.

CHRONIC MYELOGENOUS LEUKEMIA, BCR-ABL1 POSITIVE

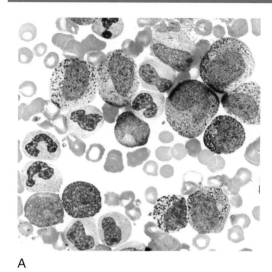

A

FIGURE 17–1A Peripheral blood. Note immature basophils and eosinophil (original size × 500).

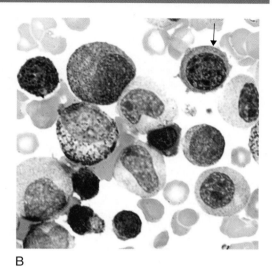

B

FIGURE 17–1B Peripheral blood. Arrow shows a micromegakaryocyte.

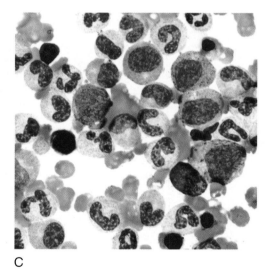

C

FIGURE 17–1C A spectrum of granulocytes, including multiple myelocytes, bands, and an immature basophil (BM × 500).

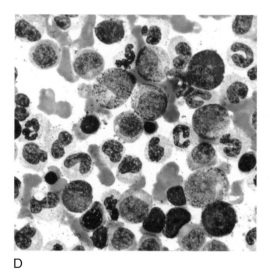

D

FIGURE 17–1D Multiple eosinophils, some of them immature (BM × 500).

NOTE: BCR-ABL positivity must be present for diagnosis.

MORPHOLOGY
Peripheral Blood: Chronic phase*
LEUKOCYTES
Marked leukocytosis (12-1000 × 10^9/L)
- Spectrum of myeloid cells with a predominance of myelocytes and segmented neutrophils
- Myeloblasts less than 5%
- ± Pseudo-Pelger-Huët cells
- Basophilia
- Eosinophilia
- ± Monocytosis
- Leukocyte alkaline phosphatase (LAP) markedly decreased (Figure 17–2)

ERYTHROCYTES
Normal or decreased in number
PLATELETS
- Normal or increased
- ± Circulating micromegakaryocytes

Bone Marrow: Chronic phase*
- Hypercellular with expansion of granulocyte pool
- Myeloid:Erythroid (M:E) ratio increased
- Myeloblasts less than 5%
- Megakaryocytes normal to increased; may be immature and/or atypical
- ± Pseudo-Gaucher cells (see Figure 22–1A)
- ± Sea blue histiocytes (see Figure 22–5A)

---

*Before development of tyrosine kinase inhibitors for treatment, CML would progress through phases, from chronic to accelerated to blast phase, with increasing numbers of blasts, basophils, micromegakaryocytes, and dysplasia. (See a hematology textbook, such as *Rodak's Hematology,* for a complete discussion of the progression of CML.)

LEUKOCYTE ALKALINE PHOSPHATASE (LAP)

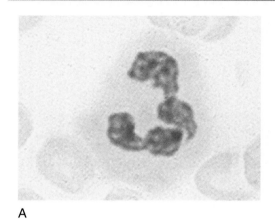

A

FIGURE 17–2A LAP-(0) (PB×1000).

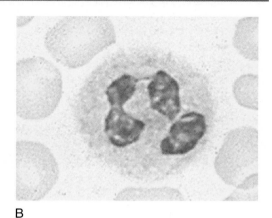

B

FIGURE 17–2B LAP (1+) (PB×1000).

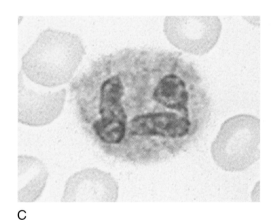

C

FIGURE 17–2C LAP (2+) (PB×1000).

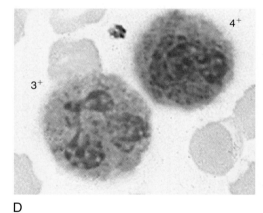

D

FIGURE 17–2D LAP (3+, 4+) (PB×1000).

LAP is an enzyme found in secondary granules of neutrophils. LAP activity is scored from 0 to 4+ in the mature segmented neutrophils and bands. One hundred cells are scored and results are added together for the LAP score. A normal score is approximately 20 to 100. Low (<20) scores may be found in untreated CML, paroxysmal nocturnal hemoglobinuria, sideroblastic anemia, and myelodysplastic syndromes. Higher scores may be found in leukemoid reactions (Table 17-2).

GENETICS
BCR-ABL positivity must be present for diagnosis.

TABLE 17-2

Comparison of Chronic Myelogenous Leukemia (CML) and Leukemoid Reaction in Peripheral Blood		
	CML	**Leukemoid Reaction***
Neutrophils	Increased with immature cells; peaks at myelocyte and segmented neutrophil stages	Increased with immature forms; orderly progression of maturation stages with no peaks
Eosinophils Basophils	Increased with immature forms	Normal
Platelets	Abnormal number Abnormal morphology	Normal
Dyspoiesis	Present	Absent, but may be reactive changes
Leukocyte alkaline phosphatase	Markedly decreased	Increased
BCR/ABL1	Positive	Negative

*Leukemoid reaction: persistent neutrophilic leukocytosis above 50,000/uL when the cause is other than leukemia.

POLYCYTHEMIA VERA

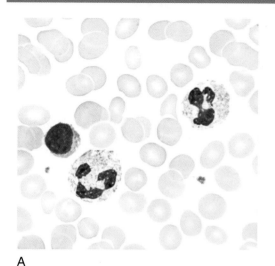

A

FIGURE 17–3A Peripheral blood (original magnification × 1000).

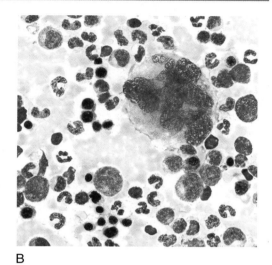

B

FIGURE 17–3B Bone marrow (original magnification × 500).

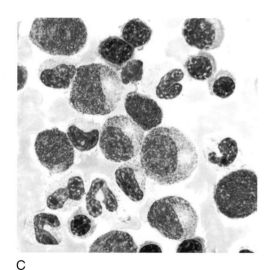

C

FIGURE 17–3C Bone marrow (original magnification × 1000).

MORPHOLOGY
Peripheral Blood:
LEUKOCYTES

Normal or increased

- Neutrophilia with few metamyelocytes, rare myelocytes
- Promyelocytes and myeloblasts extremely rare
- ± Eosinophilia and/or basophilia

ERYTHROCYTES

Absolute erythrocytosis

- Hemoglobin greater than 18.5 g/dL in male individuals
- Hemoglobin greater than 16.5 g/dL in female individuals

PLATELETS

Normal or increased

Bone Marrow:
- Hypercellular with panmyelosis
- M:E ratio usually normal
- Megakaryocytes may be abnormal in size and morphology

GENETICS
JAK2 V617F or other JAK2 mutation is found in more than 95% of cases, but is not specific for PV.

ESSENTIAL THROMBOCYTHEMIA

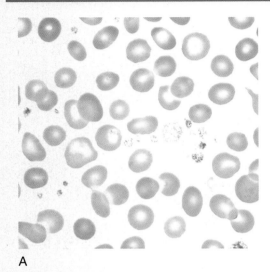

A

FIGURE 17–4A Peripheral blood (original magnification × 1000).

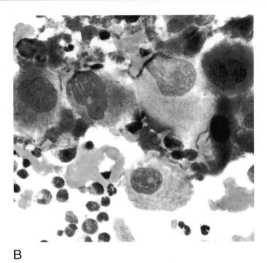

B

FIGURE 17–4B Bone marrow (original magnification × 500).

MORPHOLOGY
Peripheral Blood:

LEUKOCYTES

Normal or slightly increased

Normal maturation and distribution

ERYTHROCYTES

Normal or slightly decreased

PLATELETS

Marked sustained thrombocytosis

Variation in size from tiny to giant

Bone Marrow: Hypercellular with expansion of the megakaryocyte pool

- Large megakaryocytes with abundant cytoplasm
- May exhibit hyperlobulation

Mild granulocytic hyperplasia

Mild erythrocytic hyperplasia

GENETICS
No specific genetic or cytogenetic abnormality, but up to 50% of cases carry JAK2 V617F. JAK2 is also found in polycythemia vera and primary myelofibrosis.

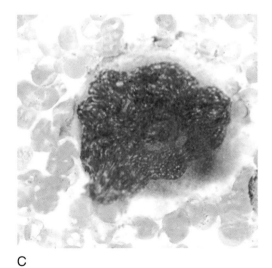

C

FIGURE 17–4C Bone marrow showing abnormal hyperlobulated megakaryocte (original magnification × 1000).

PRIMARY MYELOFIBROSIS

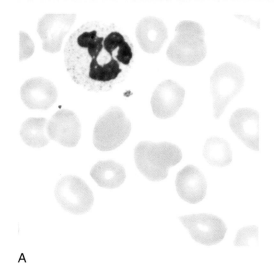

A

FIGURE 17–5A Peripheral blood (×1000; subtle changes).

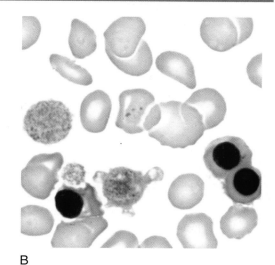

B

FIGURE 17–5B Peripheral blood (×1000; more advanced case).

MORPHOLOGY

Peripheral Blood:

LEUKOCYTES

Normal, increased, or decreased
- Immature granulocytes
- Less than 5% blasts

ERYTHROCYTES

Normal or decreased
- Teardrop cells common, nucleated erythrocytes, polychromasia

PLATELETS

Low, normal, or increased
- May be giant with atypical shapes
- Abnormal granulation
- ± Circulating micromegakaryocytes

Bone Marrow: Aspiration attempts often result in a dry tap; biopsy results exhibit marked fibrosis with islands of hematopoietic activity and pockets of clumped megakaryocytes

GENETICS

No specific genetic or cytogenetic abnormality, but up to 50% of cases carry JAK2 V617F. JAK2 is also found in polycythemia vera and essential thrombocythemia.

CHAPTER 18

MYELODYSPLASTIC SYNDROMES

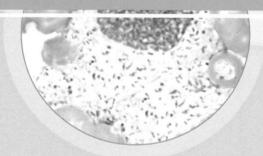

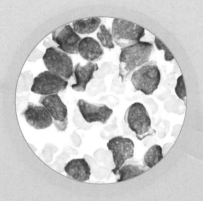

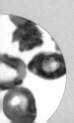

M yelodysplastic syndromes (MDSs) are acquired clonal hematological disorders characterized by normocellular/hypercellular marrow, ineffective hematopoiesis that leads to progressive cytopenia, and dysplasia in peripheral blood, reflecting maturation defects in erythrocytes, leukocytes, and/or platelets.

MDSs are heterogeneous and have a multitude of expressions; however, two morphologic findings are common to all types of MDS: the presence of progressive cytopenias in spite of a cellular bone marrow and dyspoiesis in one or more cell lines. Subtypes of the 2008 World Health Organization classification of MDSs are listed in Box 18-1.

BOX 18-1

World Health Organization Classification of Myelodysplastic Syndromes (2008)

Refractory cytopenia with unilineage dysplasia
Refractory anemia with ringed sideroblasts
Refractory cytopenia with multilineage dysplasia
Refractory anemia with excess blasts
Myelodysplastic syndrome with isolated del(5q)
Myelodysplastic syndrome, unclassifiable
Childhood myelodysplastic syndrome (provisional)

From Swerdlow SH, Campo E, Harris NL, et al (editors): *WHO classification of tumours of haematopoietic and lymphoid tissues,* ed 4, Lyon, France, IARC Press, 2008.

All photomicrographs are ×1000 original magnification with Wright-Giemsa staining unless stated otherwise.

DYSERYTHROPOIESIS

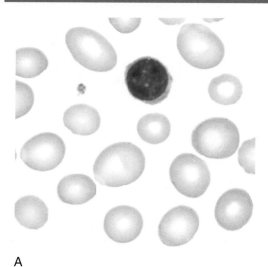

A

FIGURE 18–1A Oval macrocytes.

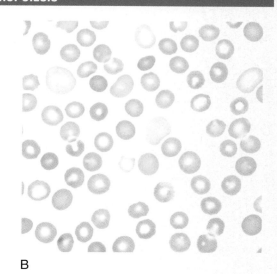

B

FIGURE 18–1B Dimorphic erythrocyte population (PB ×500).

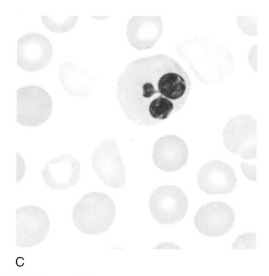

C

FIGURE 18–1C Nucleated erythrocyte with abnormal nuclear shape.

MORPHOLOGY: May include any or all of the following:

Peripheral Blood:
- Oval macrocytes
- Hypochromic microcytes
- Dimorphic erythrocyte population

Bone Marrow:
- Multinucleated erythrocyte precursors
- Abnormal nuclear shapes
- Nuclear bridging in bone marrow
- Uneven cytoplasmic staining
- Ringed sideroblasts

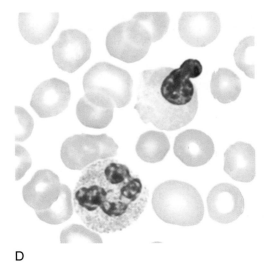

D

FIGURE 18–1D Erythrocyte precursor with partial loss of nucleus.

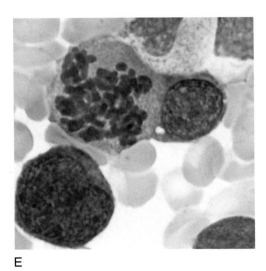

E

FIGURE 18–1E Erythrocyte precursor with abnormal nuclear shape (bilobed, with one nucleus in mitosis, demonstrating asynchrony (BM × 1000)).

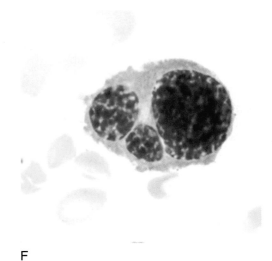

F

FIGURE 18–1F Erythrocyte precursor with three uneven nuclei (BM × 1000).

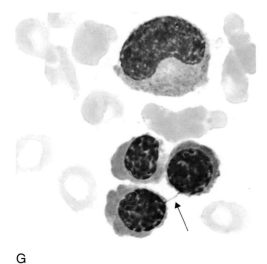

G

FIGURE 18–1G Erythrocyte precursor with nuclear bridging (*arrow*) (BM × 1000).

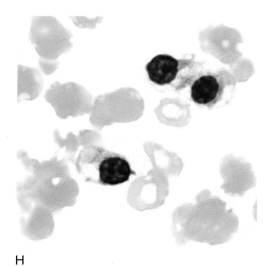

H

FIGURE 18–1H Erythrocyte precursors with uneven cytoplasmic staining (BM ×1000).

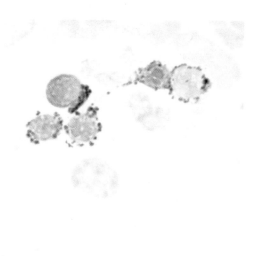

I

FIGURE 18–1I Ringed sideroblasts are precursor RBCs containing at least five iron granules that circle at least one third of the nucleus. (iron stain, BM ×1000).

DYSMYELOPOIESIS

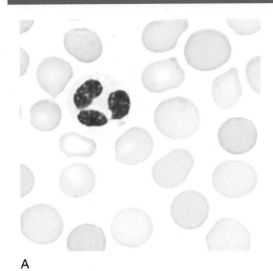

A

FIGURE 18–2A Abnormal granulation, agranular segmented neutrophil.

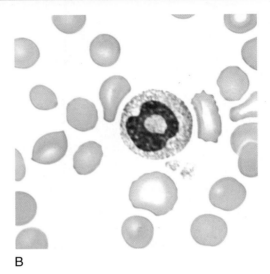

B

FIGURE 18–2B Abnormal nuclear shapes, neutrophil with circular (donut) nucleus.

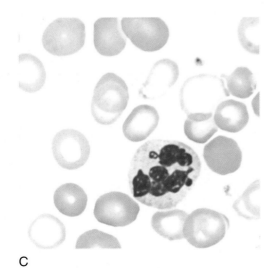

C

FIGURE 18–2C Abnormal nuclear shapes, neutrophil with hypersegmented nucleus; also exhibits hypogranulation.

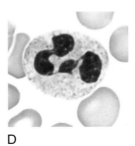

D

FIGURE 18–2D Normal neutrophil for comparison.

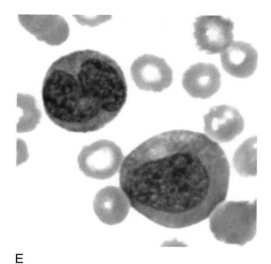

E

FIGURE 18–2E Persistent basophilic cytoplasm in abnormal myelocytes.

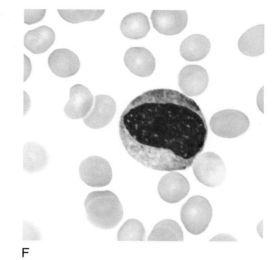

F

FIGURE 18–2F Uneven cytoplasmic staining with uneven granulation. This characteristic does not necessarily imply malignancy but is often found in MDS.

MORPHOLOGY: May include any or all of the following:

Peripheral Blood and Bone Marrow:
- Abnormal granulation
- Abnormal nuclear shapes
- Persistent basophilic cytoplasm
- Uneven cytoplasmic staining
- Pseudo-Pelger-Huët cells (see Figure 14–1)

DYSMEGAKARYOPOIESIS

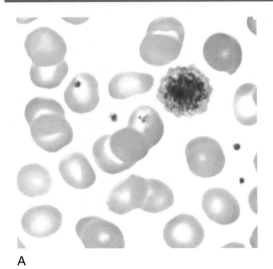

A

FIGURE 18–3A Giant platelet.

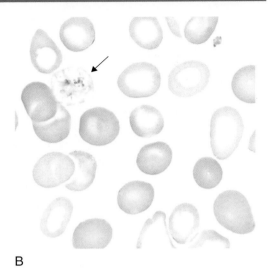

B

FIGURE 18–3B Platelet with hypogranulation.

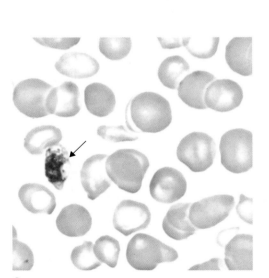

C

FIGURE 18–3C Platelet with hypergranulation.

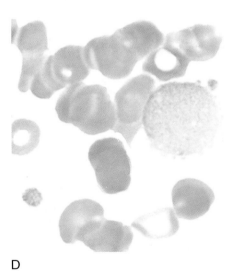

D

FIGURE 18–3D Giant platelet.

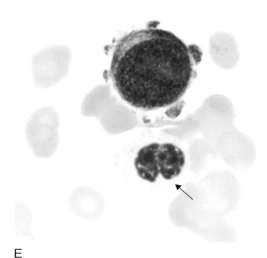

E

FIGURE 18–3E Circulating micromegakaryocyte. Hypogranular pseudo-Pelger-Huët cell at *arrow*.

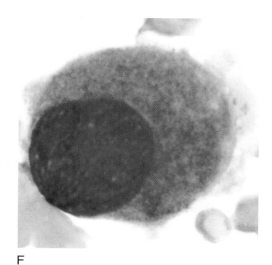

F

FIGURE 18–3F Large mononuclear megakaryocyte (BM × 1000).

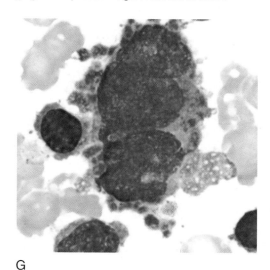

G

FIGURE 18–3G Abnormal nuclear shape, uneven number of nuclei (BM × 1000).

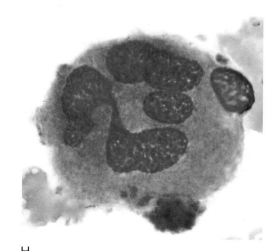

H

FIGURE 18–3H Abnormal nuclear shapes, separate nuclei (BM, original magnification × 1000).

MORPHOLOGY: May include any or all of the following:
Peripheral Blood:
- Giant platelets
- Platelets with abnormal granulation
- Circulating micromegakaryoctyes

Bone Marrow:
- Large mononuclear megakaryocytes
- Abnormal nuclear shapes
- Uneven number of nuclei
- Separate nuclei

CHAPTER 19

MATURE LYMPHOPROLIFERATIVE DISORDERS

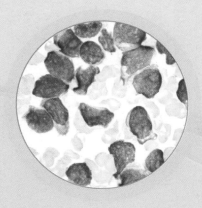

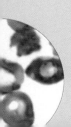

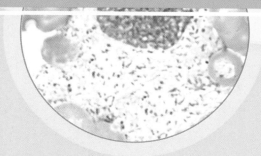

Mature lymphoproliferative disorders frequently are derived from a single clone of cells. Although this group of diseases involves lymphocytes, the morphological presentation is variable. The integration of clinical and morphological disease features with immunophenotyping is necessary for appropriate recognition and classification. Only representative samples are included in this atlas.

Note: Sustained absolute lymphocytosis in an adult should be investigated to differentiate reactive from malignant processes. Characteristics of reactive lymphocytes are listed in Appendix Table A-2.

CHRONIC LYMPHOCYTIC LEUKEMIA

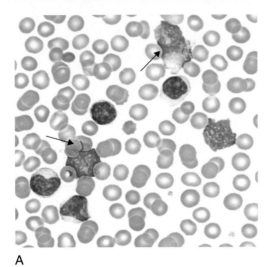

A

FIGURE 19–1A Small lymphocytes with smudge cells at arrows (PB×500).

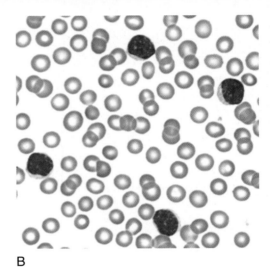

B

FIGURE 19–1B Albumin smear: same patient as presented in Figure 19–1A (PB ×500).

NOTE: Addition of albumin to blood before smear preparation stabilizes CLL cells, decreasing the formation of smudge cells and allows for accurate cell classification.

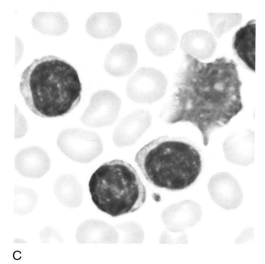

C

FIGURE 19–1C Small lymphocytes with smudge cell (PB ×1000).

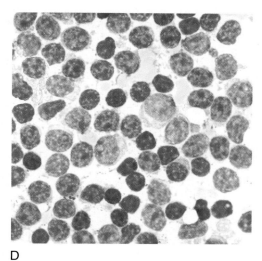

D

FIGURE 19–1D BM demonstrating many lymphocytes (BM ×500).

MORPHOLOGY

Peripheral Blood: Mature-appearing lymphocytes with round nuclei and block-type chromatin; inconspicuous nucleoli, scant cytoplasm; homogeneous appearance within a given patient; lymphocytes more fragile than normal, leading to "smudge" cells

- Absolute sustained lymphocytosis
- ± Normocytic normochromic anemia (approximately 10% of patients develop an autoimmune hemolytic anemia)
- ± Thrombocytopenia

Bone Marrow: 30% or more lymphocytes

IMMUNOPHENOTYPE

CD20[+], CD19[+], CD5[+], CD23[+]

PROLYMPHOCYTIC LEUKEMIA

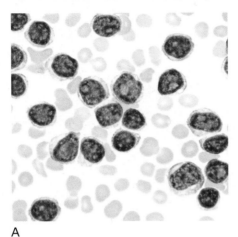

A

FIGURE 19–2A PB demonstrating many prolymphocytes with prominent nucleolus (PB ×500).

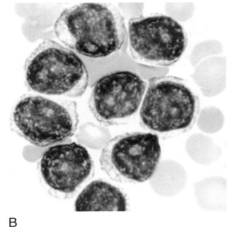

B

FIGURE 19–2B PB demonstrating prolymphocytes with prominent nucleoli (PB ×1000).

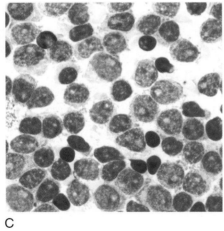

C

FIGURE 19–2C BM with many prolymphocytes (BM ×500).

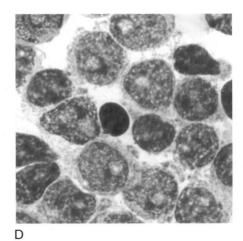

D

FIGURE 19–2D BM with many prolymphocytes (BM ×1000).

MORPHOLOGY

Peripheral Blood: Medium-sized cells (approximately twice the size of small lymphocytes), one prominent nucleolus, moderately condensed chromatin; small to moderate slightly basophilic cytoplasm

- Absolute lymphocytosis, usually greater than 100×10^9/L
- Anemia
- Thrombocytopenia

Bone Marrow: Predominantly prolymphocytes with few residual hematopoietic cells

IMMUNOPHENOTYPE

CD20$^+$, CD19$^+$, FMC7$^+$

HAIRY CELL LEUKEMIA

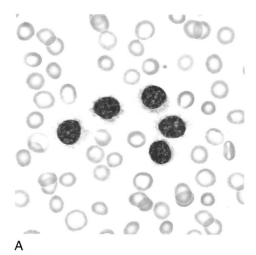

A

FIGURE 19–3A PB demonstrating hairy cells (PB ×500).

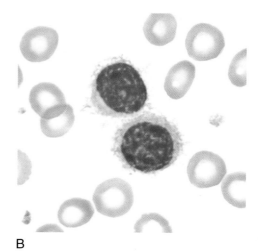

B

FIGURE 19–3B PB demonstrating hairy cells; with gray-blue hairlike projections (PB ×1000).

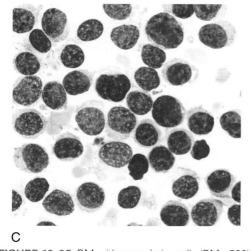

C

FIGURE 19–3C BM with many hairy cells (BM ×500).

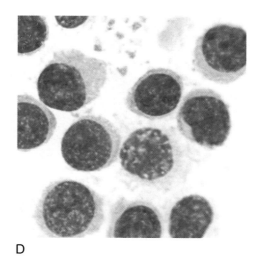

D

FIGURE 19–3D BM with many hairy cells (BM ×1000).

MORPHOLOGY

Peripheral Blood: Small- to medium-sized lymphocytes, reniform to oval nucleus with diffuse homogeneous chromatin, ± nucleolus, cytoplasm irregular with gray-blue hairlike projections
- Pancytopenia

Bone Marrow: Aspirate difficult to obtain because of marrow fibrosis (dry tap); cells more easily distinguished by phase or electron microscopy

IMMUNOPHENOTYPE

$CD19^+$, $CD20^+$, $CD22^+$, $CD11c^+$, Annexin $A1^+$

PLASMA CELL MYELOMA

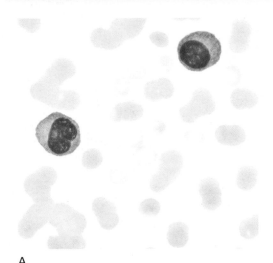

A

FIGURE 19–4A Plasma cells. Note rouleaux (PB ×500).

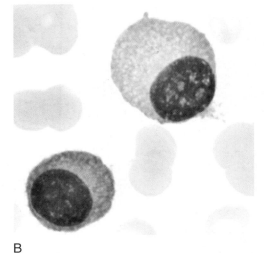

B

FIGURE 19–4B Plasma cells (PB ×1000).

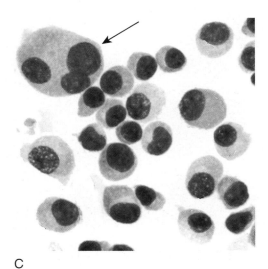

C

FIGURE 19–4C Plasma cells, one multinucleated (BM ×500).

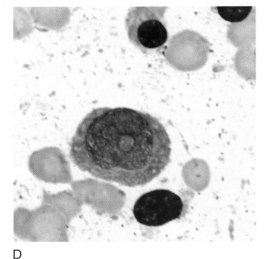

D

FIGURE 19–4D Plasmablast. with the lighter blue cytoplasm with the indistinct hof and the slightly eccentric nucleus with 2 distinct nucleoli (BM ×1000).

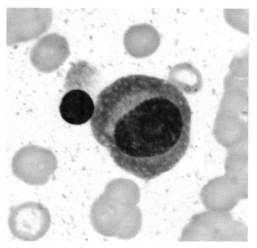

E

FIGURE 19–4E Proplasmacyte. The cytoplasm is darker blue and the perinuclear hof is distinct. The nucleus is eccentric and the nucleolus is partially masked by the clumped chromatin (PB ×1000).

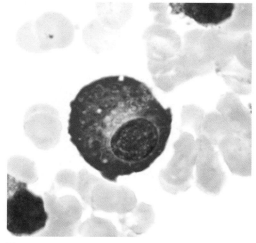

F

FIGURE 19–4F Flame cell. Associated with plasma cells that are producing immunoglobulin A (IgA) (BM ×1000).

MORPHOLOGY

Peripheral Blood: Rouleaux, rare circulating plasma cells; ± neutropenia

> **NOTE:** Greater than 2×10^9/L circulating plasma cells suggest plasma cell leukemia.

± Normocytic, normochromic anemia
± Thrombocytopenia

> **NOTE:** The background of Wright-stained blood smears may be blue due to presence of abnormal amounts of immunoglobulin.

Bone Marrow: More than 10% plasma cells, often more than 30%

Immature ± larger than normal plasma cell with increased N/C ratio; abnormal nuclear chromatin; ± nucleoli, ± multinucleated
Cytoplasm pale blue to dark blue; cytoplasm may contain immunoglobulin inclusions

IMMUNOPHENOTYPE

CD19$^-$, CD38$^+$, CD138$^+$

> **NOTE:** This disease may be distinguished from Waldenström macroglobulinemia and heavy chain disease by immunoelectrophoresis.

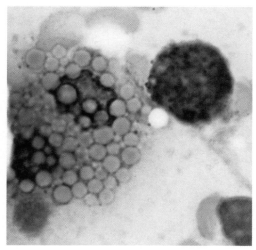

G

FIGURE 19–4G Mott cell (morula cell, grape cell). Plasma cell containing multiple round globules of immunoglobulin, which stain pink, colorless, or blue (BM ×1000).

BURKITT LEUKEMIA/LYMPHOMA

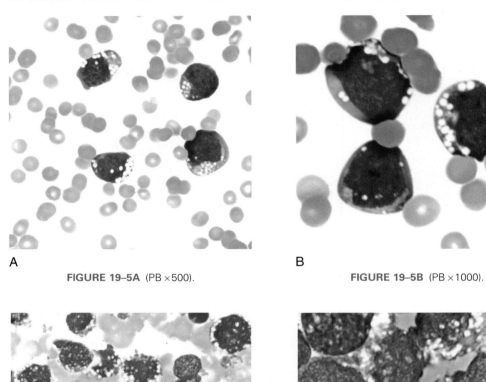

A

FIGURE 19–5A (PB ×500).

B

FIGURE 19–5B (PB ×1000).

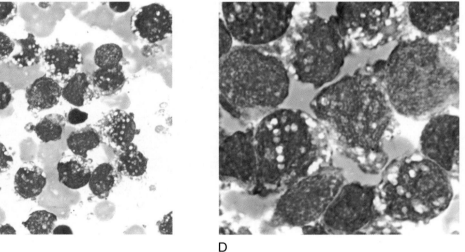

C

FIGURE 19–5C (BM ×500).

D

FIGURE 19–5D (BM ×1000).

MORPHOLOGY
Peripheral Blood: Medium- to large-sized cells with dark blue vacuolated cytoplasm, inconspicuous nucleoli
Bone Marrow: Monotonous pattern of deeply basophilic cells with vacuolated cytoplasm

IMMUNOPHENOTYPE
CD5$^-$, CD20$^+$, CD19$^+$, CD10$^+$

LYMPHOMA

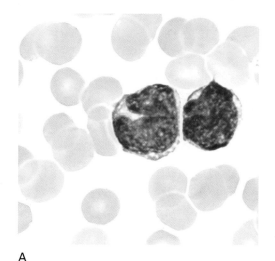

A

FIGURE 19–6A Cleaved lymphoma cells (PB ×1000).

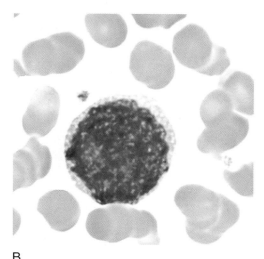

B

FIGURE 19–6B Large lymphoma cell (PB ×1000).

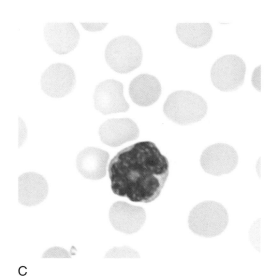

C

FIGURE 19–6C Lymphoma cell with prominent nucleoli (PB ×1000).

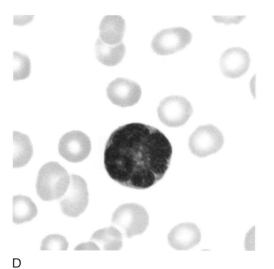

D

FIGURE 19–6D "Flower" nucleus suggestive of T-cell lymphoma (PB ×1000).

MORPHOLOGY

Peripheral Blood: Representative examples of lymphoma cells occasionally observed in peripheral blood

Bone Marrow: NA

NOTE: The diagnosis of lymphoma is determined by lymph node biopsy, immunophenotyping, and molecular genetics.

CHAPTER 20

MORPHOLOGIC CHANGES AFTER MYELOID HEMATOPOIETIC GROWTH FACTORS

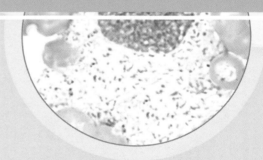

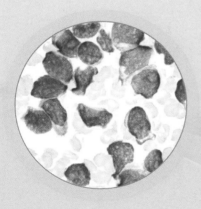

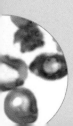

ytokine therapies, such as erythropoietin, thrombopoietin, and myeloid growth factors, such as granulocyte colony-stimulating factor (G-CSF) and granulocyte/macrophage-colony stimulating factor, are becoming common. These treatments cause characteristic changes in the peripheral blood smear. Although erythropoietin and thrombopoietin rarely create diagnostic challenges, the morphologic changes in the myeloid cell line may mimic severe infection, acute myeloid leukemia, or myelodysplastic or myeloproliferative neoplasm. Specific changes include transient leukocytosis with immature granulocytic cells, vacuolated and giant neutrophils, toxic granulation, Döhle bodies, hypogranulation, nucleated red blood cells, and as many as 5% blasts in the peripheral blood.*

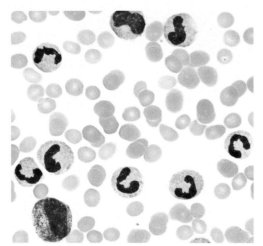

FIGURE 20–1 Leukocytosis in response to G-CSF (PB ×500).

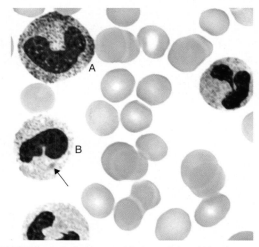

FIGURE 20–2 A, Neutrophils in peripheral blood exhibiting toxic granulation and hypogranulation. **B,** A Döhle body is present at the *arrow.*

---

*Heerema-McKenney A, Arber DA: Acute myeloid leukemia. In: Hsi ED (Editor): *Hematopathology.* In: Goldblum JR (Series Editor): *Foundations in Diagnostic Pathology,* ed 2. Philadelphia: Elsevier/Saunders, 2012, p. 419–456.

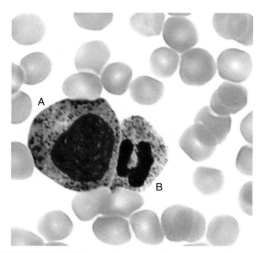

FIGURE 20–3 A, Immature asynchronous granulocyte. **B,** Mature neutrophil with toxic granulation.

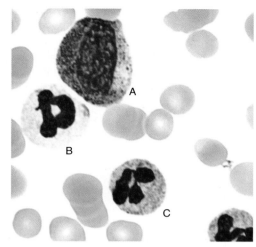

FIGURE 20–4 A, Giant asynchronous immature granulocyte. **B,** Hypogranular neutrophil with a Döhle body. **C,** Granulocyte with normal granulation.

CHAPTER 21

MICROORGANISMS

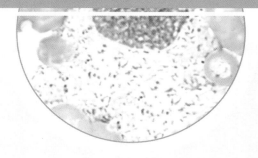

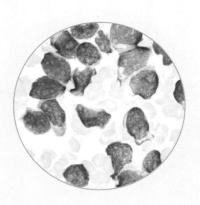

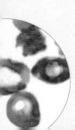

PLASMODIUM SPECIES

The following examples are representative of the developmental stages of malaria that can be seen in the peripheral blood. Detailed criteria for identification of species may be found in a parasitology text.

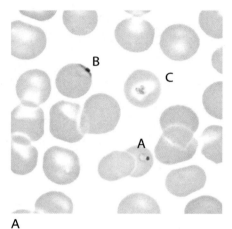

A

FIGURE 21–1A *Plasmodium* species. Rings A, applique form B and platelet on RBC C (PB × 1000). Platelets on top of RBC often have a halo, or clear area surrounding the platelet.

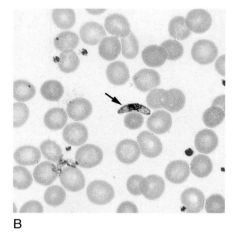

B

FIGURE 21–1B *Plasmodium falciparum* crescent (banana-shaped) gametocyte in thin peripheral blood film. (PB × 1000).
(Courtesy of Indiana Pathology Images.)

C

FIGURE 21–1C *Plasmodium vivax* schizont in a thin peripheral blood film. Note the number of merozoites and the presence of brown hemozoin pigment.
(Courtesy of Indiana Pathology Images.)

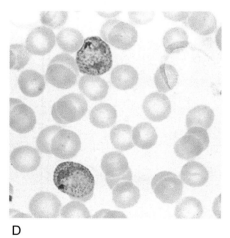

D

FIGURE 21–1D Two *Plasmodium vivax* trophozoites in a thin peripheral blood film. Note that the infected red blood cells are enlarged and contain Schüffner stippling, and the trophozoites are large and ameboid in appearance, (PB × 1000).
(Keohane EM, Smith LJ, Walenga JM: *Rodak's hematology*, ed 5, St. Louis, Elsevier, 2016.)

BABESIA SPECIES

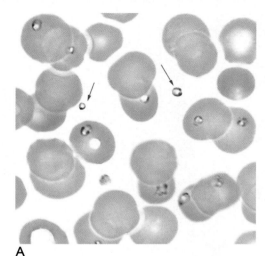

A

FIGURE 21–2A *Babesia microti* (PB ×1000).

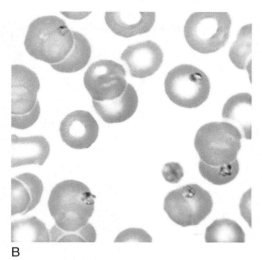

B

FIGURE 21-2B *Babesia microti* (PB ×1000).

DESCRIPTION: *Babesia* species may be confused morphologically with *Plasmodium falciparum*, but lack of pigment and absence of life cycle stages help differentiate *Babesia* spp. from *P. falciparum*. Extracellular organisms (Figure 21–2, arrows) are more often seen in *Babesia* spp. Travel history is the best way to differentiate between *Babesia* and *Plasmodium*.

LOA LOA

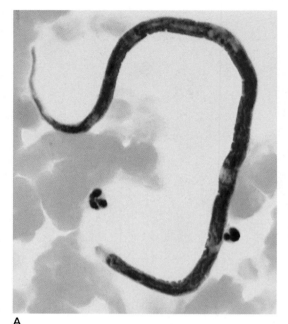

A

FIGURE 21–3A *Loa loa,* a microfilaria (PB, original magnification ×1000).

DESCRIPTION: *Loa loa* is a microfilaria (Figure 21–3). Other microfilariae may be seen in the peripheral blood. Differentiation of microfilariae may be challenging. Consult a parasitology/microbiology text, such as Mahon and Lehman's Textbook of Diagnostic Microbiology, 5e.

TRYPANOSOMES

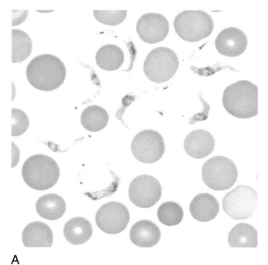

A

FIGURE 21–4A *Trypanosoma brucei gambiense* (Giemsa stain, PB ×1000).

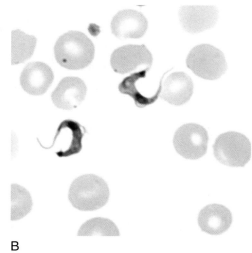

B

FIGURE 21–4B *Trypanosoma cruzi* (Giemsa stain, PB ×1000).

DESCRIPTION: Trypanosomes are examples of hemoflagellates that may occasionally be encountered in the peripheral blood (Figure 21–4A and B). Differentiating features may be found in a parasitology text.

FUNGI

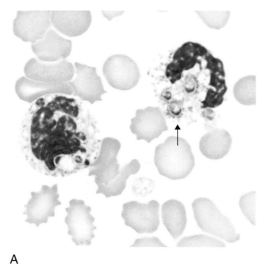

A

FIGURE 21–5A *Histoplasma capsulatum* in neutrophil (PB ×1000).

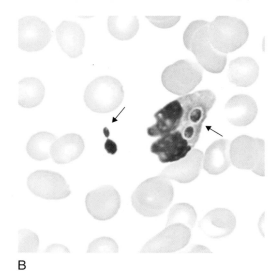

B

FIGURE 21–5B Intracellular and extracellular yeast in peripheral blood of an immunocompromised patient (PB ×1000).

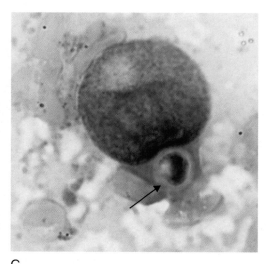

C

FIGURE 21–5C *Cryptococcus neoformans* (BM ×1000) (see also Figure 24–14).

BACTERIA

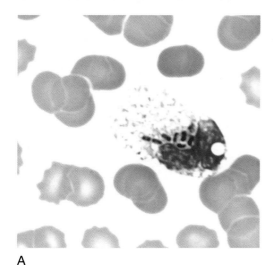

A

FIGURE 21–6A Bacilli engulfed by a leukocyte. Note vacuoles (PB ×1000).

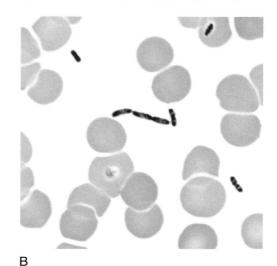

B

FIGURE 21–6B Extracellular bacteria from same specimen as Figure 21–6A. Extracellular bacteria alone may indicate contamination. Presence of intracellular bacteria may rule out contamination (PB ×1000).

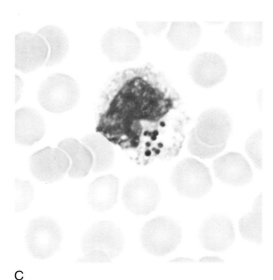

C

FIGURE 21–6C Cocci engulfed by a monocyte (PB ×1000).

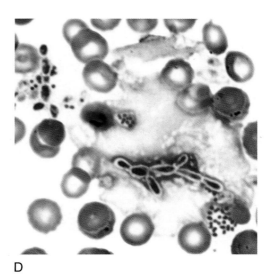

D

FIGURE 21–6D Multiple organisms, including yeast and cocci, most likely contamination from an intravenous line (PB ×1000).

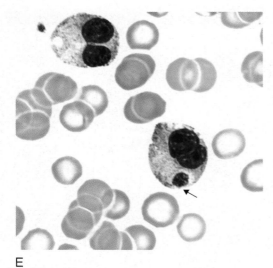

E

FIGURE 21–6E *Anaplasma phagocytophilum* in a neutrophil (PB ×1000).

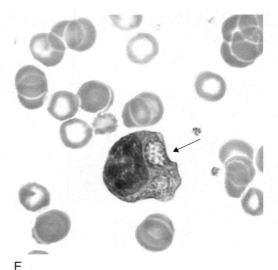

F

FIGURE 21–6F *Ehrlichia chaffeensis* in a monocyte (PB×1000).
(Courtesy J. Stephen Dumler, MD, Division of Medical Microbiology, The Johns Hopkins Medical Institutions, Baltimore, MD.)

CHAPTER 22

MISCELLANEOUS CELLS

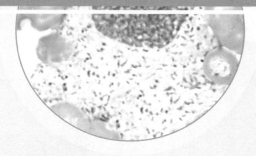

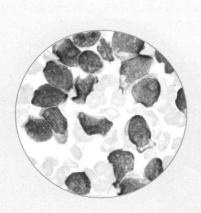

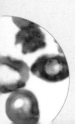

HEMATOLOGIC MANIFESTATIONS OF SYSTEMIC DISORDERS

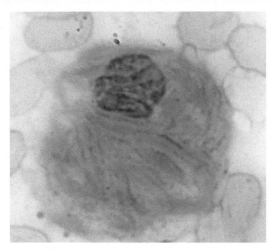

FIGURE 22–1 Gaucher cell (BM × 1000).

DESCRIPTION: The Gaucher cell is a macrophage 20 to 80 μm in diameter, with one or more small, round to oval eccentric nuclei; cytoplasm has crumpled tissue-paper appearance; found in bone marrow, spleen, liver, and other affected tissue. Engulfed material is glucocerebroside.

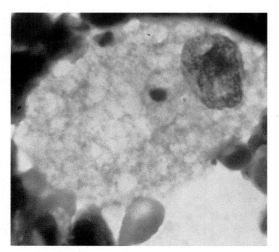

FIGURE 22–2 Niemann-Pick cell (BM × 1000).

DESCRIPTION: The Niemann-Pick cell is a macrophage, 20 to 90 μm in diameter, with a small eccentric nucleus and foamy cytoplasm. It is found in bone marrow and lymphoid tissue. The peripheral blood of patients with Niemann-Pick disease may exhibit vacuolated lymphocytes. Engulfed material is sphingomyelin.

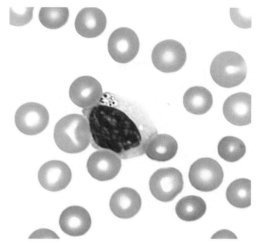

FIGURE 22–3 Lymphocyte from Sanfilippo syndrome (PB ×1000).

DESCRIPTION: Peripheral blood lymphocytes containing azurophilic granules occasionally surrounded by halos

ASSOCIATED WITH: Mucopolysaccharide storage disorders

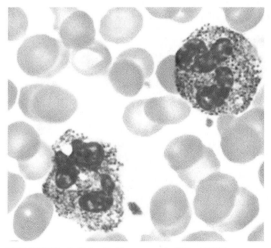

FIGURE 22–4 Alder-Reilly anomaly (PB ×1000).
(Courtesy Dennis P. O'Malley, MD, Clarient, Inc., Aliso Viejo, CA.)

DESCRIPTION: Deep purple to lilac granules difficult to distinguish from toxic granulation; occur in neutrophils and occasionally eosinophils and basophils

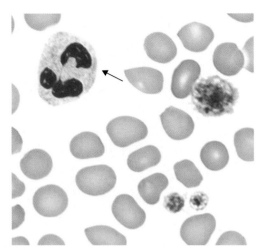

FIGURE 22–5 May-Hegglin anomaly with Döhle-like body at *arrow* (PB × 1000).

DESCRIPTION: Characterized by thrombocytopenia with large platelets and large basophilic inclusions resembling Döhle bodies in granulocytes and monocytes with the absence of toxic granulation

NOTE: These inclusions are sporadically visible by light microscopy, but always detectable by electron microscopy. The ultrastructure varies from that of Döhle bodies.

CHEDIAK HIGASHI SYNDROME

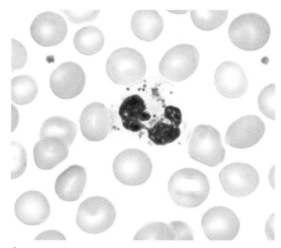

A

FIGURE 22–6A Chédiak-Higashi anomaly neutrophil with granules (PB ×1000).

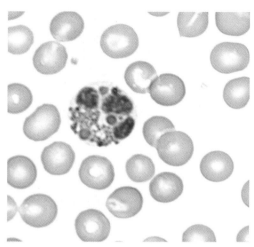

B

FIGURE 22–6B Chédiak-Higashi anomaly eosinophil with granules (PB ×1000).

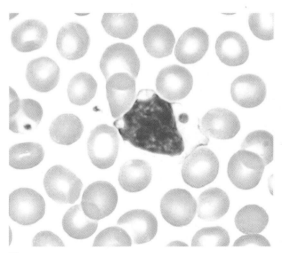

C

FIGURE 22–6C Chédiak-Higashi anomaly lymphocyte with granule (PB ×1000).

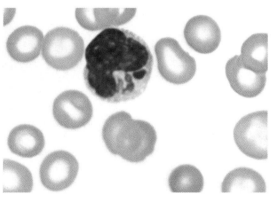

D

FIGURE 22–6D Chédiak-Higashi anomaly monocyte with granules (PB ×1000).

DESCRIPTION: Large gray-blue granules in the cytoplasm of many granulocytes. Monocytes, lymphocytes, and eosinophils may contain large red-purple granules

OTHER CELLS SEEN IN BONE MARROW

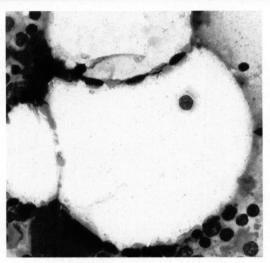

FIGURE 22–7 Fat/adipose cell (BM ×500).

DESCRIPTION: Large round cell, 50 to 80 μm; cytoplasm filled with one or several large fat vacuoles, colorless to pale blue; nucleus small, round to oval, and eccentric; chromatin coarse; nucleoli seldom seen

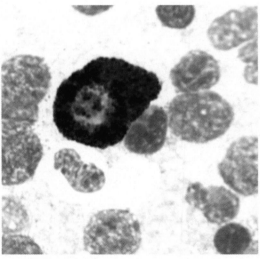

FIGURE 22–8 Mast cell (BM ×1000).

DESCRIPTION: Large cell (12 to 25 μm) with round to oval nucleus; cytoplasm is colorless to lavender with many dark blue to black granules that may partially obscure the nucleus. Constitute less than 1% of bone marrow cells. Increased numbers may be seen in allergic inflammation and anaphylaxis

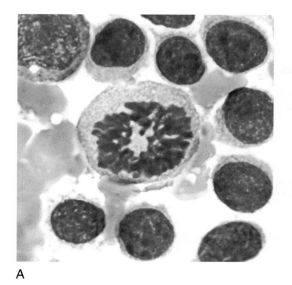

A

FIGURE 22–9A Mitosis (BM ×1000).

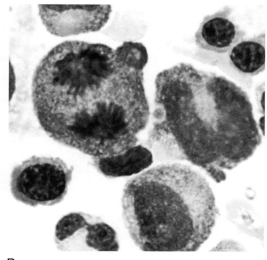

B

FIGURE 22–9B Mitosis (BM ×1000).

DESCRIPTION: Mitotic figure: a cell that is dividing. Increased numbers may be seen in neoplastic disorders

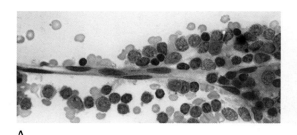

A

FIGURE 22–10A Endothelial cells lining a blood vessel (BM, original magnification ×500).

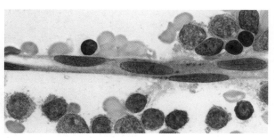

B

FIGURE 22–10B Endothelial cells (BM, original magnification ×1000).

DESCRIPTION: Large, elongated cells, 20 to 30 μm; one oval nucleus with dense chromatin; nucleoli not visible; function is to line blood vessels; rarely seen in peripheral blood

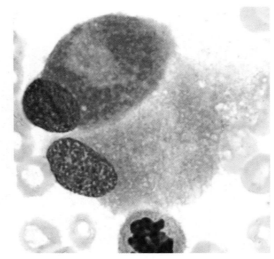

FIGURE 22–11 Osteoblasts (BM, original magnification ×1000).

DESCRIPTION: Large comet or tadpole-shaped cell, 30 μm; single, round, eccentrically placed nucleus, may be partially extruded; abundant cytoplasm with chromophobic area located away from nucleus; often appears in groups; function in synthesis of bone

NOTE: May be confused with plasma cells (see Figure 19-4B).

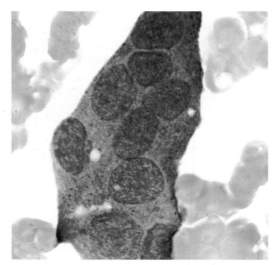

FIGURE 22–12 Osteoclast (BM, original magnification × 1000).

DESCRIPTION: Very large (>100 μm), multinucleated with irregularly shaped ruffled border; nuclei are round to oval, separate and distinct with little variation in nuclear size; cytoplasm may vary from slightly basophilic to very acidophilic; coarse granules may be present; osteoclasts function in the resorption of bone

NOTE: May be confused with megakaryocytes (see Figure 4-6A).

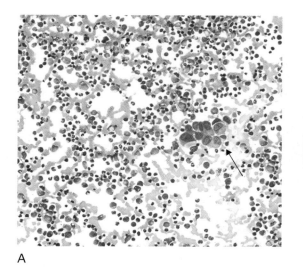

A

FIGURE 22–13A Metastatic tumor (BM ×100).

FIGURE 22–13B Metastatic tumor (BM ×500).

B

DESCRIPTION: Tumor cell clusters may be recognized during the ×100 scan of bone marrow, especially at or near the edge of the coverslip or glass slide. Characteristics of the tumor cells are more easily observed at ×1000 magnification. Cells are variable in size and shape within the same tumor clump. Nuclei vary in size and staining characteristics. Nucleoli are usually visible. It is sometimes difficult to distinguish one cell from another because of "molding" of cells

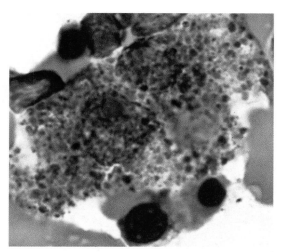

FIGURE 22–14 Sea blue histiocyte (BM ×1000).

DESCRIPTION: Macrophage 20 to 60 μm in diameter with eccentric nucleus; cytoplasm contains varying numbers of prominent blue-green granules; may be seen in diseases with rapid cell turnover, such as myeloproliferative neoplasms

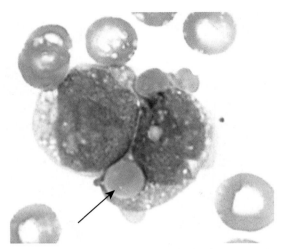

FIGURE 22–15 Erythrophagocytosis (BM × 1000).

DESCRIPTION: Monocyte or macrophage with engulfed erythrocyte at *arrow*; may be seen in some transfusion reactions

ARTIFACTS IN PERIPHERAL BLOOD SMEARS

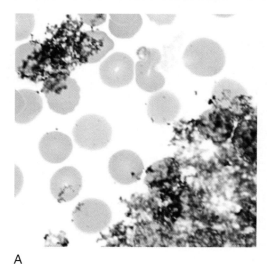

A

FIGURE 22–16A Precipitated stain (PB ×1000).

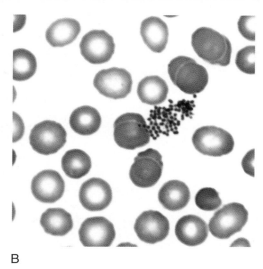

B

FIGURE 22–16B Bacteria in peripheral blood for comparison with precipitated stain (PB ×1000).

DESCRIPTION: Precipitate is in focus, but the cells are not. If bacteria are present within a cell, both cell and bacteria should be in focus at the same time

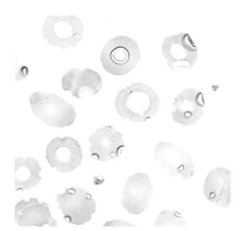

FIGURE 22–17 Drying artifact in RBCs (PB ×1000).

DESCRIPTION: Highly refractile areas because of slow drying of blood film

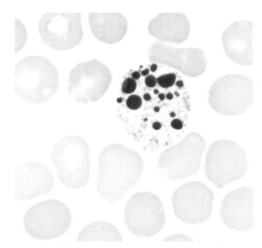

FIGURE 22–18 Necrotic cell (PB ×1000).

DESCRIPTION: Nuclear degeneration observe lack of chromatin pattern and nuclear filaments

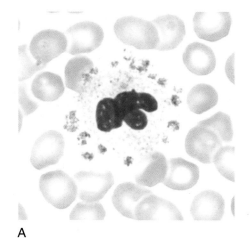

A

FIGURE 22–19A Platelet satellitism (PB ×1000).

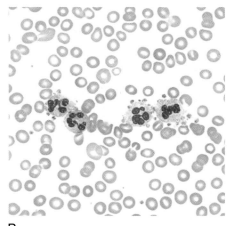

B

FIGURE 22–19B Platelet satellitism (PB ×500).

DESCRIPTION: Platelets adhering to neutrophils; in vitro phenomenon in blood collected in ethylenediaminetetraacetic acid (EDTA) in rare individuals, which may cause falsely decreased platelet counts. May be resolved by collecting blood in sodium citrate*

---

*Keohane EA, Smith L, Walenga J, eds: *Rodak's Hematology: Clinical Principles and Applications*, ed 5, Philadelphia, Saunders/Elsevier, 2016.

CHAPTER 23

NORMAL NEWBORN PERIPHERAL BLOOD MORPHOLOGY

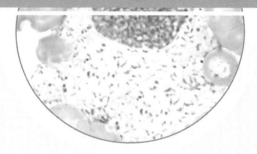

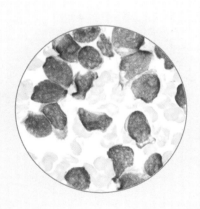

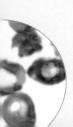

n the healthy full-term newborn, peripheral blood collected within the first 12 hours of birth has a distinctive morphology. Some morphological changes persist for 3 to 5 days after birth. These changes should be recognized as physiological and not pathological. For a fuller discussion of hematology in the newborn, refer to a hematology textbook, such as *Rodak's Hematology: Clinical Principles and Applications,*[*] or a pediatric hematology text, such as *Nathan and Oski's Hematology of Infancy and Childhood.*[†]

Entire books have been written to address abnormal hematology in neonates and especially in the premature infant. This chapter does not attempt to address those disorders but rather depicts morphological changes commonly seen in the healthy newborn.

Erythrocyte morphology demonstrates macrocytes, with a mean cell volume of 119 ± 9.4 fL at birth, which declines dramatically after the first 12 hours. Around 3 to 10 orthochromic normoblasts (nucleated red blood cells) may be seen per 100 white blood cells and should disappear by day 5. Polychromasia reflects the erythropoietic activity of the newborn. Anisocytosis is reflected in the red blood cell distribution width index, which ranges from 14.2% to 17.8%.

Occasional spherocytes are common, varying from one every two fields to one or more in every field.

Newborn total leukocyte counts are higher than for adults, and newborns have more segmented and band neutrophils than at any other time in childhood.[‡] An occasional metamyelocyte may be seen without evidence of infection. Monocyte morphology is similar to that of the adult.

Lymphocyte morphology is pleomorphic, spanning the range from reactive to mature. The presence of a nucleolus is not uncommon; however, the chromatin pattern is coarse and not as fine as seen in blasts. Hematogones (immature B cells) are occasionally seen in bone marrow and peripheral blood of newborns. Caution must be exercised to correctly differentiate hematogones from blasts that may indicate a pathologic condition.

[*]Keohane EM, Smith LJ, Walenga JM (editors): *Rodak's Hematology: Clinical Principles and Applications,* ed 5, St. Louis, Elsevier/Saunders, 2016.

[†]Orkin SH, Nathan DG, Ginsburg D et al: *Nathan and Oski's Hematology and Oncology of Infancy and Childhood,* ed 8, Philadelphia, Elsevier/Saunders, 2016.

[‡]Ambruso DR, Nuss R, Wang M: Hematologic Disorders. In: *Current Diagnosis & Treatment: Pediatrics, 22e.* New York, NY, McGraw-Hill, 2014.

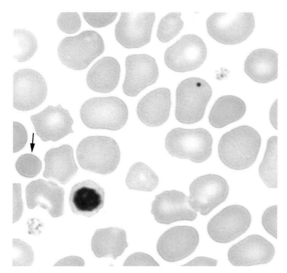

FIGURE 23–1 Peripheral blood from a neonate demonstrating macrocytes, polychromasia, nucleated red blood cell, Howell-Jolly body, and one spherocyte (*arrow*) (PB ×1000).

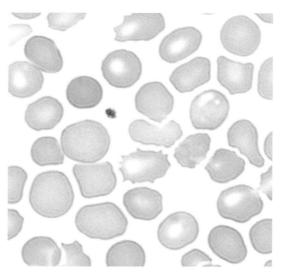

FIGURE 23–2 Peripheral blood from a neonate demonstrating polychromasia, anisocytosis, echinocytes, and spherocytes (PB ×1000).

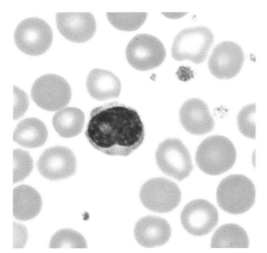

FIGURE 23–3 Lymphocyte from neonate blood. Although there appears to be a nucleolus, the chromatin pattern is coarse (PB ×1000).

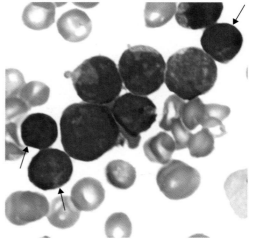

FIGURE 23–4 Bone marrow from neonate with acute lymphoblastic leukemia, demonstrating hematogones and lymphoblasts. Hematogones vary in size. Nucleus is round to oval with condensed, smudged chromatin. Nucleoli are absent or indistinct. Cytoplasm is indiscernible to scant. *Arrows* point to hematogones. Most of the other cells are blasts (BM ×1000). See Chapter 16 for comparison with blasts.

CHAPTER 24

BODY FLUIDS

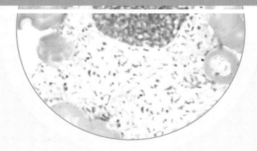

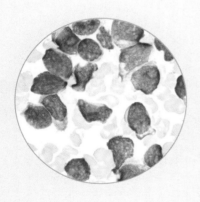

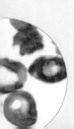

Fluid in the cavities that surround organs may serve as a lubricant or shock absorber, enable the circulation of nutrients, or function for the collection of waste. Evaluation of body fluids may include total volume, gross appearance, total cell count, differential cell count, identification of crystals, biochemical analysis, microbiological examination, immunological studies, and cytological examination. The most common body fluid specimens received in the laboratory are cerebrospinal fluid (CSF); pleural, peritoneal, and pericardial fluids (together known as *serous* fluids); and synovial fluids. Under normal circumstances, the only fluid that is present in an amount large enough to sample is CSF. Therefore, when other fluids are present in detectable amounts, disease is suspected.

This atlas addresses primarily the elements of fluids that are observable through a microscope. For a more detailed explanation of body fluids, consult a hematology or urinalysis textbook that includes a discussion of body fluids, such as *Rodak's Hematology: Clinical Principles and Applications*[*] or *Fundamentals of Urine and Body Fluid Analysis.*[†]

Because the number of cells in fluids is often very small, a concentrated specimen is preferable for performing the morphological examination. Preparation of slides using a cytocentrifuge is the method commonly used. This centrifuge spins at a low speed to minimize distortion of cells, concentrating the cells into a "button" on a small area of the glass slide. Slide preparation requires cytofunnel, filter paper to absorb excess fluid, and a glass slide. These elements are joined together in a clip assembly, and the entire apparatus is then centrifuged slowly. Excess fluid is absorbed by the filter paper, leaving a monolayer of cells in a small button on the slide. When the cytospin slide is removed from the centrifuge, it should be dry. If the cell button is still wet, the centrifugation time may need to be extended.

When preparing cytocentrifuge slides, a consistent amount of fluid should be used to generate a consistent yield of cells. Usually two to six drops of fluid are used depending on the nucleated cell count. Five drops of fluid will generally yield enough cells to perform a 100-cell differential if the nucleated cell count is at least $3/mm^3$. For very high counts, a dilution with normal saline may be made. The area of the slide where the cell button will be deposited should be marked with a wax pencil in case the number of cells recovered is small and difficult to locate (Figure 24–1). Alternatively, specially marked slides can be used.

There may be some distortion of cells as a result of centrifugation or when cell counts are high. Dilutions with normal saline should be made before centrifugation to minimize distortion when nucleated cell counts are high. When the red blood cell (RBC) count is extremely high (more than 1 million/mm^3), the slide should be made in the same manner as the peripheral blood smear slide (see Chapter 1). However, the examination of the smear should be performed at the end of the slide rather than the battlement pattern used for blood smears.

---

[*]Keohane EM, Smith LJ, Walenga JM, (editors): *Rodak's Hematology: Clinical Principles and Applications,* ed 5, St. Louis, Elsevier/Saunders, 2016.

[†]Brunzel NA: *Fundamentals of Urine and Body Fluid Analysis,* ed 3, St. Louis, Elsevier/Saunders, 2012.

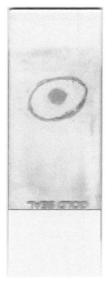

A

FIGURE 24–1A Wright-stained cytocentrifuge slide demonstrating a concentrated button of cells within the marked circle.

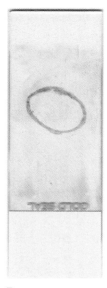

B

FIGURE 24–1B Wright-stained cytocentrifuge slide from a cerebrospinal fluid containing few cells, demonstrating the importance of marking the cell concentration area.

This is because the larger, and usually more significant, cells are likely to be pushed to the end of the slide.

When examining the cytospin slide, the entire cell button should be scanned under the 10× objective to search for the presence of tumor cells. The 50× or 100× oil immersion lens should be used to differentiate the white blood cells. For the performance of the differential, any area of the cell button may be used. If the cell count is low, a systematic pattern, starting at one end of the side of the button and working toward the other, is recommended.

Any cell that is seen in the peripheral blood may be found in a body fluid in addition to cells specific to that fluid (e.g., mesothelial cells, macrophages, tumor cells). However, the cells look somewhat different than in peripheral blood, and some in vitro degeneration is normal. The presence of organisms, such as yeast and bacteria, should also be noted (see Figures 24–12 to 24–14).

CELLS COMMONLY SEEN IN CEREBROSPINAL FLUID

FIGURE 24–2 Segmented neutrophils (CSF × 1000).

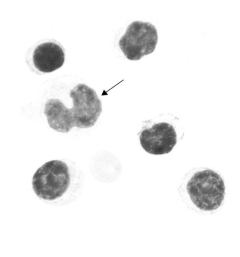

FIGURE 24–3 Lymphocytes and monocyte (*arrow*) (CSF × 1000).

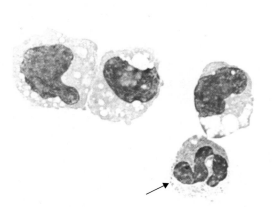

FIGURE 24–4 Monocytes and segmented neutrophil (*arrow*) (CSF × 1000).

COMMENTS: Small numbers of neutrophils, lymphocytes, and monocytes may be seen in normal CSF.

Increased numbers of neutrophils are associated with bacterial meningitis; early stages of viral, fungal, and tubercular meningitis; intracranial hemorrhage; intrathecal injections; central nervous system (CNS) infarct; malignancy; or abscess.

Increased numbers of lymphocytes and monocytes are associated with viral, fungal, tubercular, and bacterial meningitis and multiple sclerosis.

CELLS SOMETIMES FOUND IN CEREBROSPINAL FLUID

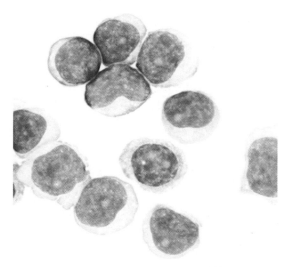

FIGURE 24–5 Reactive lymphocytes (CSF × 1000).

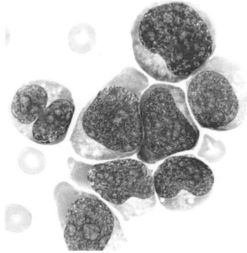

FIGURE 24–6 Acute lymphoblastic leukemia (CSF × 1000).

Reactive lymphocytes (Figure 24–5) are associated with viral meningitis and other antigenic stimulation. The cells will vary in size; nuclear shape may be irregular and cytoplasm may be scant to abundant with pale to intense staining characteristics. (See description of reactive lymphocytes, Figure 14–7.)

Blasts in the CSF may have some of the characteristics of the acute lymphoblastic leukemia (ALL) blasts seen in the peripheral blood (Figure 24–6; see Chapter 16). It is not unusual for ALL to have CNS involvement, and blasts may be present in the CSF before being observed in the peripheral blood.

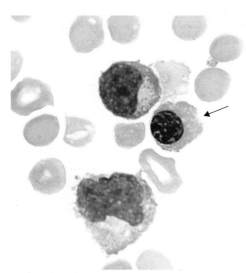

FIGURE 24–7 Nucleated red blood cell (CSF × 1000).

ASSOCIATED WITH: Traumatic lumbar tap in premature infants, blood dyscrasias with circulating nucleated RBCs, and bone marrow contamination of CSF

CELLS SOMETIMES FOUND IN CEREBROSPINAL FLUID AFTER CENTRAL NERVOUS SYSTEM HEMORRHAGE

The following sequence of events is a typical reaction to intracranial hemorrhage or repeated lumbar punctures:

1. Neutrophils and macrophages: appear within 2 to 4 hours
2. Erythrophages: identifiable from 1 to 7 days
3. Hemosiderin and siderophages: observable from 2 days to 2 months
4. Hematoidin crystals: recognizable in 2 to 4 weeks.

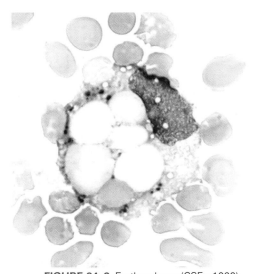

FIGURE 24–8 Erythrophage (CSF × 1000).

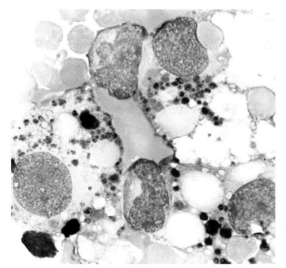

FIGURE 24–9 Hemosiderin (CSF × 1000).

Macrophage with engulfed RBCs. RBCs are digested by enzymatic activity within the macrophage. The digestive process causes the RBCs to lose color and to appear as vacuoles within the cytoplasm of some macrophages.

Blue to black granules that contain iron, resulting from the degradation of hemoglobin, may be present in CSF for up to 2 months after intracranial hemorrhage. The cellular inclusions can be positively identified with an iron stain.

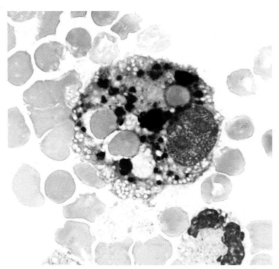

FIGURE 24–10 Siderophage (CSF ×1000).

Macrophage containing hemosiderin.

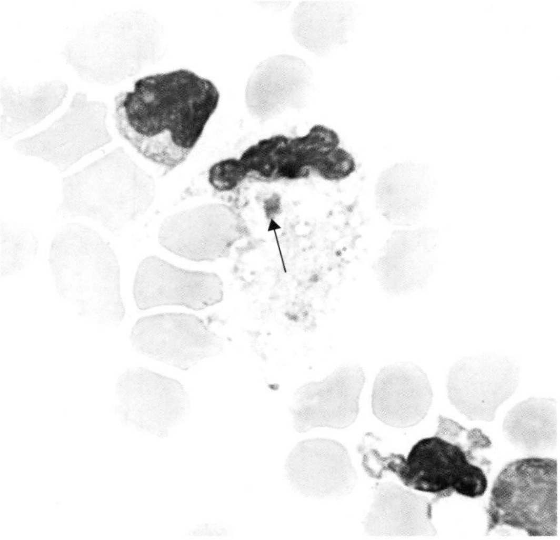

FIGURE 24–11 Hematoidin within macrophage (*arrow*) (CSF ×1000).

Gold intracellular crystals composed of bilirubin. Hematoidin is the result of the catabolism of hemoglobin and may be present for several weeks after CNS hemorrhage.

NOTE: Macrophages may display the presence of a variety of particles within one cell. For example, one macrophage may contain hemosiderin and hematoidin.

ORGANISMS SOMETIMES FOUND IN CEREBROSPINAL FLUID

CSF is a sterile body fluid. The following are examples of some organisms that have been seen in CSF, but it is far from an all-inclusive list of possibilities (Figures 24–12 to 24–14). Note that organisms may be intracellular, extracellular, or both.

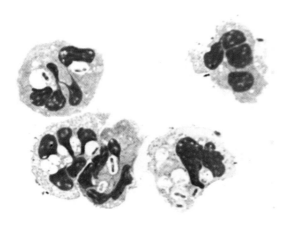

FIGURE 24–12 Bacteria engulfed by neutrophils (CSF ×1000).

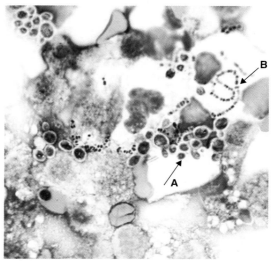

FIGURE 24–13 *Histoplasma capsulatum A* within macrophage (CSF ×1000). Note the presence of bacteria in chains B.

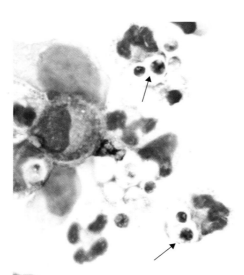

FIGURE 24–14 *Cryptococcus neoformans* inside neutrophil (CSF ×1000).

CELLS SOMETIMES FOUND IN SEROUS BODY FLUIDS
(PLEURAL, PERICARDIAL, AND PERITONEAL)

NOTE: Any of the cell types found in the peripheral blood may be found in serous fluids.

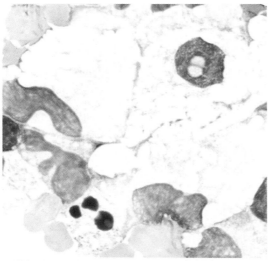

FIGURE 24–15 Macrophages (pleural fluid × 1000).

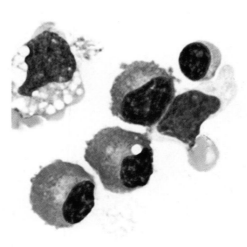

FIGURE 24–16 Plasma cells (pleural fluid × 1000).

DESCRIPTION: Large cells with eccentric nuclei and vacuolated cytoplasm may be present in all body fluids. They may be seen with or without inclusions, such as RBCs, siderotic granules, or lipids.

DESCRIPTION: Round to oval cell with eccentric nuclei, dark blue cytoplasm, perinuclear hof 8 to 29 μm in diameter

ASSOCIATED WITH: Rheumatoid arthritis, malignancy, tuberculosis, and other conditions that exhibit lymphocytosis

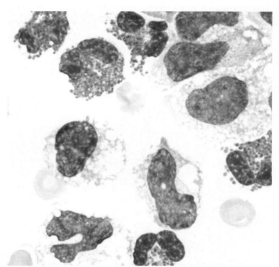

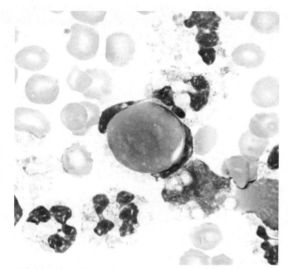

FIGURE 24–17 Eosinophils and macrophages (pleural fluid × 1000).

FIGURE 24–18 Lupus erythematosus cell (pleural fluid × 1000).

ASSOCIATED WITH: Allergic reaction, air and/or foreign matter within the body cavity, parasites

Intact neutrophil with engulfed homogeneous mass. The mass displaces the nucleus of the neutrophil and is composed of degenerated nuclear material. Lupus erythematosus (LE) cells are formed in vivo and in vitro in serous fluids. LE cells may also form in synovial fluids.

ASSOCIATED WITH: Lupus erythematosus

MESOTHELIAL CELLS

Mesothelial cells are shed from membranes that line body cavities and are often found in serous fluids.

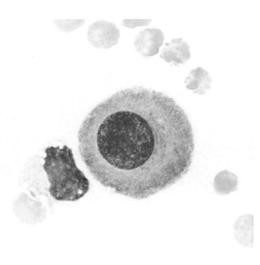

FIGURE 24–19 Mesothelial cell with pale blue cytoplasm (pleural fluid ×1000).

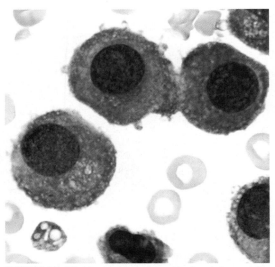

FIGURE 24–20 Mesothelial cells with deeply basophilic cytoplasm (pleural fluid ×1000).

MORPHOLOGY:

SHAPE: Pleomorphic

SIZE: 12 to 30 μm

NUCLEUS: Round to oval with smooth nuclear borders; nucleus may be eccentric or multinucleated, making the distinction between the mesothelial and plasma cell difficult at times
Nucleoli: 1 to 3, uniform in size and shape
Chromatin: Fine, evenly distributed

CYTOPLASM: Abundant, light gray to deeply basophilic
Vacuoles: Occasional

NOTE: Mesothelial cells may appear as single cells in clumps or sheets. The clumping of cells together and the variability of appearance require careful observation to accurately differentiate mesothelial cells from malignant cells. Three characteristics can aid in this determination:

1. Mesothelial cells on a smear tend to be similar to one another.
2. The nuclear membrane appears smooth by light microscopy.
3. Mesothelial cells maintain cytoplasmic borders. When appearing in clumps, there may be clear spaces between the cells. These spaces are often referred to as "windows."

MULTINUCLEATED MESOTHELIAL CELLS

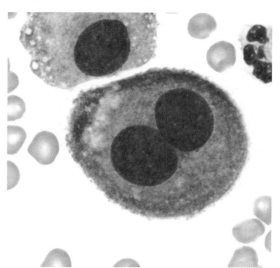

FIGURE 24–21 Binucleated mesothelial cell (pleural fluid × 1000).

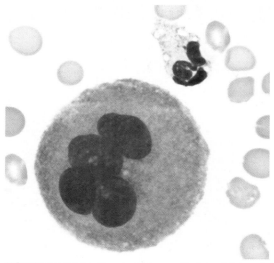

FIGURE 24–22 Multinucleated mesothelial cell (pleural fluid × 1000).

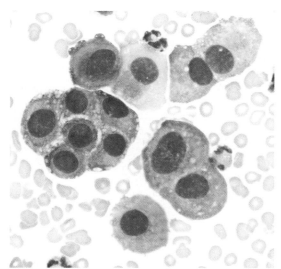

FIGURE 24–23 Clump of mesothelial cells. Note "windows" in the large clump (pleural fluid × 500).

TABLE 24–1

Characteristics of Benign and Malignant Cells

Benign	Malignant
Occasional large cells	Many cells may be very large
Light to dark staining	May be very basophilic
Rare mitotic figures	May have several mitotic figures
Round to oval nucleus; nuclei are uniform size with varying amounts of cytoplasm	May have irregular or jagged nuclear shape
Nuclear edge is smooth	Edges of nucleus may be indistinct and irregular
Nucleus intact	Nucleus may be disintegrated at edges
Nucleoli are small, if present	Nucleoli may be large and prominent
In multinuclear cells (mesothelial), all nuclei have similar appearance (size and shape)	Multinuclear cells have varying sizes and shapes of nuclei
Moderate to small N:C* ratio	May have high N:C ratio
Clumps of cells have similar appearance among cells, are on the same plane of focus, and may have "windows" between cells	Clumps of cells contain cells of varying sizes and shapes, are "three-dimensional" (have to focus up and down to see all cells), and have dark staining borders. No "windows" between cells

From: Keohane EM, Smith LJ, Walenga JM (editors): *Rodak's Hematology: Clinical Principles and Applications,* ed 5, St. Louis Elsevier/ Saunders, 2016.
*N:C, nuclear:cytoplasmic.

It is not always possible to distinguish malignant cells from mesothelial cells with the use of solely the light microscope. The following criteria for malignant cells may aid in this distinction.

NUCLEUS: High N:C ratio, membrane irregular
Nucleoli: Multiple, large with irregular staining
Chromatin: Hyperchromatic with uneven distribution

CYTOPLASM: Irregular membrane

NOTE: Smears with cells displaying one or more of the above characteristics should be referred to a qualified cytopathologist for confirmation. See Table 24–1 for a comparison of benign and malignant features. Malignant cells tend to form clumps with cytoplasmic molding. The boundaries between cells may be indistinguishable.

MALIGNANT CELLS SOMETIMES SEEN IN SEROUS FLUIDS

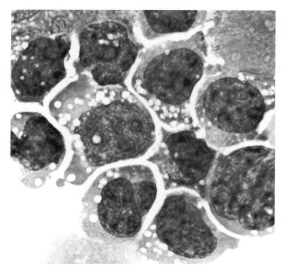

FIGURE 24–24 Non-Hodgkin lymphoma (pleural fluid × 1000).

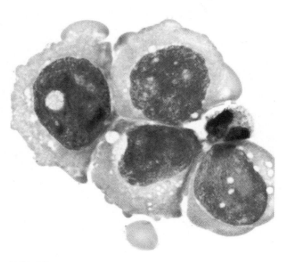

FIGURE 24–25 Breast tumor metastases (pleural fluid × 1000).

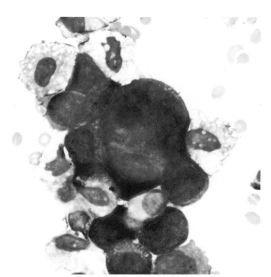

FIGURE 24–26 Malignant tumor (pleural fluid × 500). Note molding of cytoplasm (no "windows" between cells).

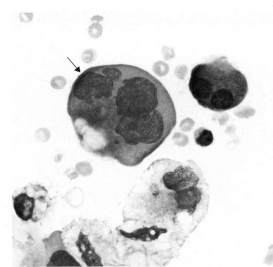

FIGURE 24–27 Adenocarcinoma, metastases from uterine cancer (pleural fluid ×500). Note irregular nuclear membranes.

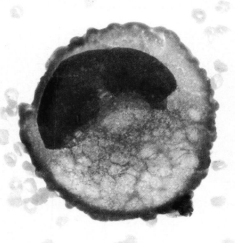

FIGURE 24–28 Malignant tumor (pleural fluid ×500).

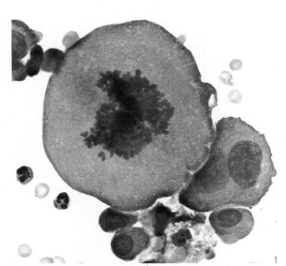

FIGURE 24–29 Mitotic figure in malignancy (pleural fluid ×500).

Mitotic figures may be found in normal fluids and are not necessarily an indication of malignancy. The size of this mitotic figure, however, is quite large, and malignant cells were easily found.

CRYSTALS SOMETIMES FOUND IN SYNOVIAL FLUID

Cells that may be found in normal synovial fluids include lymphocytes, monocytes, and synovial cells. Synovial cells, which line the synovial cavity, resemble mesothelial cells (see Figure 24–19) but are smaller and less numerous. Increased numbers of polymorphonuclear neutrophils may be seen in bacterial infection and acute inflammation. When neutrophils are seen, a careful search for bacteria should be performed. Tumor cells are possible but quite rare. LE cells may also be seen (see Figure 24–18).

Each evaluation of synovial fluid should include a careful examination for crystals. Although it is not necessary to use a stain, Wright stain is sometimes used. A polarizing microscope with a red compensator should always be used for confirmation. The most common crystals are monosodium urate, calcium pyrophosphate dihydrate, and cholesterol.

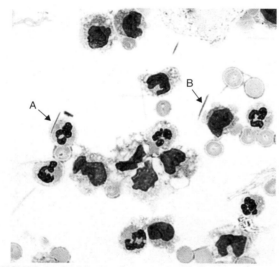

FIGURE 24–30 Monosodium urate crystals (synovial fluid ×1000; Wright stain). Needlelike crystals with pointed ends may be intracellular A, extracellular B, or both.

ASSOCIATED WITH: Gout

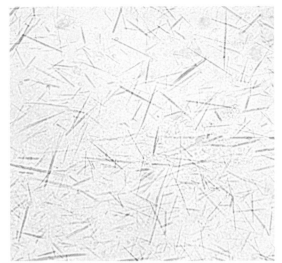

FIGURE 24–31 Monosodium urate crystals (synovial
fluid ×1000; unstained).
(Courtesy George Girgis, MT [ASCP], Indiana University
Health.)

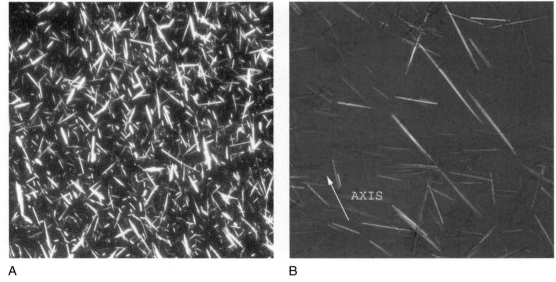

A   B

FIGURE 24–32 Monosodium urate crystals, polarized light microscopy **(A)** and with red compensator **(B)** (synovial
fluid ×1000).
(Courtesy George Girgis, MT [ASCP], Indiana University Health.)

Notice the orientation of the crystals and corresponding colors. Crystals appear yellow when parallel to the axis
of slow vibration and blue when perpendicular to the axis.

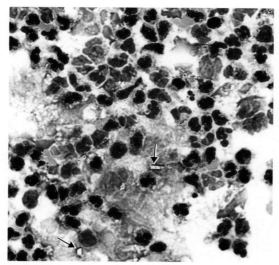

FIGURE 24–33 Calcium pyrophosphate dihydrate crystals (synovial fluid × 1000; Wright stain).

Rhomboid, rod-like chunky crystals may be intracellular, extracellular, or both.

ASSOCIATED WITH: Pseudogout or pyrophosphate gout

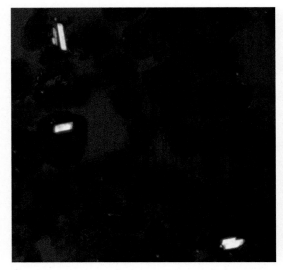

A

FIGURE 24–34A Calcium pyrophosphate dihydrate crystals, polarized light microscopy (synovial fluid ×1000). (Courtesy George Girgis, MT [ASCP], Indiana University Health.)

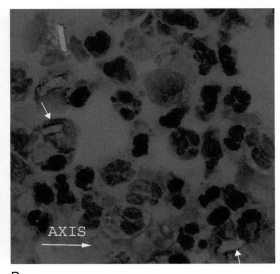

B

FIGURE 24–34B Calcium pyrophosphate dihydrate crystals, polarized with red compensator (synovial fluid ×1000). (Courtesy George Girgis, MT [ASCP], Indiana University Health.)

Notice the orientation of the crystals and corresponding colors. Crystals appear blue when parallel to the axis of slow vibration and yellow when perpendicular to the axis. Calcium pyrophosphate dihydrate is only weakly birefringent, so that the colors are not as bright as monosodium urate crystals (see Figure 24–32).

FIGURE 24–35 Cholesterol crystals (synovial fluid ×500; unstained).

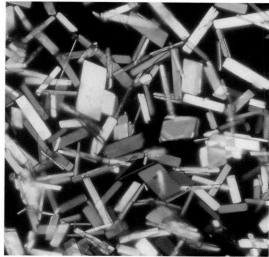

FIGURE 24–36 Cholesterol crystals (synovial fluid ×500; polarized light microscopy).
(Courtesy George Girgis, MT [ASCP], Indiana University Health.)

Large, flat rectangular plates with notched corners.

ASSOCIATED WITH: Chronic inflammatory conditions and considered a nonspecific finding

NOTE: It is necessary to use polarized light for confirmation of cholesterol crystals, but it is not necessary to use a red compensator.

OTHER STRUCTURES SOMETIMES SEEN IN BODY FLUIDS

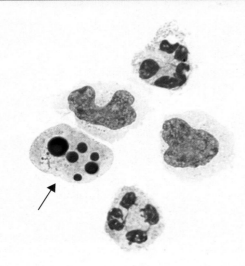

FIGURE 24–37 Necrosis (pleural fluid ×500).

Intracellular nuclear degeneration appearing as darkly stained mass(es) (*arrow*), compared with two segmented neutrophils. Contrary to necrosis seen in peripheral blood, necrotic figures in body fluids can develop in vivo.

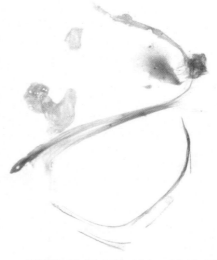

FIGURE 24–38 Artifact (pleural fluid ×500).

Fibers from the filter paper may appear near the edges of the slide. Fibers may be birefringent but lack the sharp pointed ends of monosodium urate crystals.

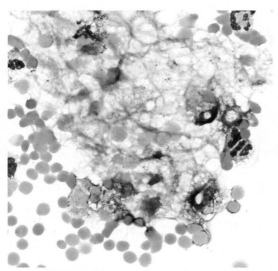

FIGURE 24–39 Brain tissue (CSF ×500).

The specimen in Figure 24–39 is from a patient who experienced head trauma.

a-βeta-lipoproteinemia Autosomal recessive disorder of lipoprotein metabolism. Characterized by the presence of peripheral blood film acanthocytes, and low plasma cholesterol levels.

abscess Accumulation of pus within a body tissue.

acanthocyte Red blood cell with spiny projections of varying lengths distributed irregularly over its surface; usually dense, lacking central pallor. Associated with lipid imbalance. Contrast with the echinocyte, which has regular projections of uniform length.

acanthocytosis Presence of acanthocytes in the blood. Associated with abetalipoproteinemia or abnormalities of lipid metabolism, such as abnormalities occurring in liver disease.

acute Describes diseases whose symptoms begin abruptly with marked intensity and then subside after a relatively short period.

acute leukemia Malignant, unregulated proliferation of hematopoietic progenitors of the myeloid or lymphoid cell lines. Characterized by abrupt onset of symptoms, and if left untreated, death occurs within months of the time of diagnosis.

adenopathy Enlargement of one or more lymph nodes.

adipocyte Fat cell; adipocytes make up adipose tissue and the yellow portion of the bone marrow.

adipose Fat.

agglutination Cross-linking of antigen-bearing cells or particles by a specific antibody to form visible clumps.

aggregation Cluster or clump of similar cell types or particles; for example, attachment of platelets to other platelets, red blood cell clumping.

agranular Without granules.

agranulocytosis Any condition involving markedly decreased numbers of granulocytes (segmented neutrophils, or band neutrophils).

Alder-Reilly anomaly Autosomal dominant polysaccharide metabolism disorder in which white blood cells (WBCs) of the myelocytic series, and sometimes all WBCs, contain coarse azurophilic mucopolysaccharide granules.

alloimmune Producing antibodies to antigens derived from a genetically dissimilar individual of the same species.

alloimmune hemolytic anemia Anemia caused by antibodies that are stimulated by exposure to foreign red blood cell (RBC) antigens. Antibodies coat and shorten the life span of circulating RBCs. This is the basis for hemolytic disease of the fetus and newborn.

α-thalassemia Moderate to severe inherited anemia caused by a decreased or absent production of the α-globin chains of hemoglobin.

amyloidosis Disease in which a waxy, starchlike glycoprotein (amyloid) accumulates in tissues and organs, impairing their function.

anemia Diminished delivery of oxygen to tissues, as evidenced by pallor, malaise, and dyspnea. May be caused by blood loss, decreased red blood cell (RBC) production, and increased RBC destruction (shortened life span).

anisocytosis Abnormal red blood cell (RBC) morphology characterized by considerable variation in RBC volume or RBC diameter on a blood film.

anoxia Inadequate tissue oxygenation caused by poor lung perfusion or a diminished blood supply.

antibody (Ab) Specialized protein (immunoglobulin) that is produced by B lymphocytes and plasma cells when the immune system is exposed to foreign antigens from bacteria, viruses, or other biologic materials.

antigen Molecule that the immune system recognizes as foreign and that subsequently evokes an immune response.

aplasia Failure of the normal process of cell generation and development. Bone marrow aplasia is the loss of all bone marrow cellular elements.

aplastic anemia Deficiency of all of the formed elements of blood, representing a failure of the blood cell generating capacity of bone marrow.

artifact Something not naturally present, especially when introduced by an external source.

asynchrony Disturbance of coordination that causes processes to occur at abnormal times. In hematopoietic cell development, a difference in rate between cytoplasmic and nuclear maturation.

atypical lymphocytes See reactive lymphocyte.

Aüer rod Abnormal needle-shaped, or round pink to purple inclusion in the cytoplasm of myeloblasts and promyelocytes; composed of condensed primary granules. Indicates acute myeloid leukemia.

autoantibody Antibody produced by an individual that recognizes and binds an antigen on the individual's own tissues.

autoimmune Describes an immune response in which an antibody forms to one's own tissues.

autoimmune hemolytic anemia Anemia characterized by premature red blood cell (RBC) destruction. Autoantibodies to the RBC surface antigens bind the membrane causing rapid splenic clearance and hemolysis.

azurophilic Having cellular structures that stain blue with Giemsa stain and red–purple with Wright stain.

azurophilic granules Primary cytoplasmic granules in myelocytic cells, which when stained with Wright stain appear reddish purple. Azurophilic granules of different composition may also appear in a minority of lymphocytes.

B cell Any of a family of lymphocytes that produce antibodies. The end product of B cell maturation is the plasma cell.

Babesia Protozoal parasite transmitted by ticks that infects human red blood cells and causes babesiosis, a malaria-like illness. The parasite is an intracellular ringlike structure 2 to 3 μm in diameter. Extracellular organisms may also be seen; this is a helpful characteristic in differentiating Babesia from Plasmodium falciparum in which extracellular ring forms are not usually seen.

band neutrophil (band) Immediate precursor of the mature segmented neutrophil. Band neutrophils have a nonsegmented, usually curved nucleus, and are present in the bone marrow and peripheral blood.

Bart hemoglobin Deletion of all alpha genes in the hemoglobin molecule (Υ_4). Associated with hydrops fetalis syndrome.

basophil (baso) Granulocytic white blood cell characterized by cytoplasmic granules that stain bluish black when exposed to a basic dye. Cytoplasmic granules of basophils are of variable size and may obscure the nucleus.

basophilia Refers to an increase in basophils in the blood. Also causes a diffuse bluish tinge throughout cytoplasm.

basophilic normoblast (prorubricyte) Second identifiable stage in bone marrow erythrocytic maturation; it is derived from the pronormoblast (rubriblast). Typically 10 to 15 μm in diameter, the basophilic normoblast (prorubricyte) has cytoplasm that stains dark blue with Wright stain.

basophilic stippling Barely visible dark blue to purple granules evenly distributed within a red blood cell stained with Wright stain. Composed of precipitated ribosomal protein and RNA.

benign Noncancerous or nonmalignant.

β-thalassemia Inherited anemia caused by diminished synthesis of the β-globin chains of hemoglobin.

bilirubin Gold-red-brown pigment, the main component of bile and a major metabolic product of the heme portion of hemoglobin, released from senescent red blood cells.

birefringent Having two different refractive indices. A crystal that is birefringent appears bright against a black background.

blast Earliest, least differentiated stage of hematopoietic maturation that can be identified by its morphology in a Wright-stained bone marrow smear; for example, myeloblast, pronormoblast (rubriblast), and lymphoblast.

bone marrow Gelatinous red and yellow tissue filling the medullary cavities of bones. Red marrow is found in most bones of infants and children; also in the ends of long bones and the cavities of flat bones in adults.

bone marrow aspirate specimen A 1 to 1.5-mL aliquot of gelatinous red marrow obtained by passing a needle into the marrow cavity and applying negative pressure. The aspirate specimen is spread as a smear on a microscope slide, stained, and examined for hematologic or systemic disease. The aspirate specimen provides for analysis of individual cell morphology.

bone marrow biopsy specimen A 1 to 2 cm cylinder of gelatinous red marrow obtained by passing a biopsy cannula into the marrow cavity, rotating, and withdrawing. The cylinder is fixed in formalin, sectioned, stained, and examined for hematologic or systemic disease. The biopsy specimen provides for analysis of bone marrow architecture.

Burkitt lymphoma Lymphatic solid tissue tumor composed of mature B lymphocytes, with a characteristic morphology called Burkitt cells. Burkitt cells appear in lymph node biopsies, bone marrow, and occasionally in peripheral blood, and have dark blue cytoplasm with multiple vacuoles creating a "starry sky" pattern.

burr cell See echinocyte

burst-forming unit (BFU) Early hematopoietic progenitor cell stages of the erythroid and megakaryocytic cell lines characterized by their tissue culture growth pattern in which large colonies are produced. Contrast with the more differentiated colony-forming units, which produce smaller colonies.

Cabot rings Threadlike structures that appear as purple-blue loops or rings in Wright-stained red blood cells. They are remnants of mitotic spindle fibers that indicate hematologic disease such as megaloblastic or refractory anemia.

cell membrane Cell surface composed of two layers of phospholipids intermixed with cholesterol and a variety of specialized glycoproteins that support cell structure, signaling, and ion transport.

centriole Cylindrical organelle composed of microtubules. Two centrioles typically orient perpendicular to each other forming the centrosome, located near the nucleus.

cerebrospinal fluid (CSF) Fluid that flows through and protects the four ventricles of the brain, the subarachnoid spaces, and the spinal canal. CSF is derived from plasma and is the site of bacterial and viral infections called meningitis or encephalitis. CSF is sampled by lumbar puncture.

CFU–GEMM Colony Forming Unit-Granulocyte, Erythrocyte, Monocyte, Megakaryocyte.

Chédiak–Higashi anomaly Autosomal recessive disorder characterized by partial albinism, photophobia, susceptibility to infection, and the presence of giant large gray-blue granules in the cytoplasm of Wright-stained granulocytes and monocytes. Lymphocytes and eosinophils may contain large red-purple granules.

chemotherapy Use of medicine or drugs to treat cancer.

chromatin The material composed in the chromosomes of organisms other than bacteria (i.e., eukaryotes). It consists of protein, RNA, and DNA.

chronic Persisting over a long period of time, often for the remainder of a person's life.

chronic leukemia Malignant, unregulated proliferation of myeloid or lymphoid cells that appear at several stages of differentiation in peripheral blood. Characterized by slow onset and progression of symptoms.

clone Group of genetically identical cells derived from a single common cell through mitosis.

cluster of differentiation (CD) Cell surface membrane receptors or markers used to characterize cells by their functions. CD profiles are used in flow cytometry to identify cell types. CDs are used in hematology to identify cell clones associated with lymphoid and myeloid leukemias and lymphomas.

codocyte (target cell) Poorly hemoglobinized red blood cell (RBC) that appears in hemoglobinopathies, thalassemia, and liver disease. In a Wright-stained peripheral blood film, hemoglobin concentrates in the center of the RBC and around the periphery causing the cell to resemble a "bull's-eye."

cold agglutinin IgM autoantibody specific for red blood cell surface membrane antigens usually of the Ii system that typically reacts at temperatures below 30° C. Commonly found in healthy adults.

cold agglutinin disease Acquired autoimmune hemolytic anemia resulting from red blood cell (RBC) agglutination by IgM autoantibodies that react with RBCs at temperatures above 30° C.

colony-forming unit (CFU) Hematopoietic progenitor cells that are derived from the pluripotential hematopoietic stem cell, and give rise to the different cell lineages of the bone marrow. Named because of their ability to form colonies in tissue culture.

colony-forming unit–granulocyte, erythrocyte, monocyte, and megakaryocyte (CFU–GEMM) Hematopoietic progenitor cell capable of differentiating into the granulocytic (myelocytic), erythrocytic (normoblastic), monocytic, or megakaryocytic cell lines.

colony-stimulating factor (CSF) Cytokine that promotes the division and differentiation of hematopoietic cells.

cytocentrifuge a centrifuge used for depositing cells suspended in a liquid onto a slide for microscopic examination. Often used in preparation for body fluid examination.

cytochemical analysis Use of specialized stains to detect cellular enzymes and other chemicals in peripheral blood films and bone marrow aspirate smears. May be used to differentiate hematologic diseases, especially leukemias.

cytogenetics Branch of genetics devoted to the laboratory study of visible chromosome abnormalities, such as deletions, translocations, and aneuploidy.

cytokines Cellular products that influence the function or activity of other cells. Cytokines include colony-stimulating factors, interferons, interleukins, and lymphokines. Also referred to as growth factors.

cytopenia Reduced cell count in one or more of any blood cell line: red blood cells, white blood cells, or platelets.

dacryocyte (teardrop cell) Red blood cell with a single pointed extension, resembling a teardrop. Dacryocytes are often seen in the extramedullary hematopoiesis, such as primary myelofibrosis and megaloblastic anemia

deoxyribonucleic acid (DNA) Double-stranded, helical nucleic acid that carries genetic information. DNA is composed of nucleotide sequences with four repeating bases: adenine, cytosine, guanine, and thymine. During mitosis DNA condenses to form chromosomes.

differential white blood cell count Review and tabulation of 100 to 200 white blood cells (WBCs) in a stained blood film. The different types of WBCs are counted and reported as absolute counts or percentages of total WBCs. In automated hematology analyzers, the differential WBC count is accomplished by counting thousands of WBCs using various technologies.

dimorphic Occurring in two distinct forms that differ in one or more characteristics, such as coloration, size, or shape.

disseminated intravascular coagulation (DIC) Uncontrolled activation of thrombin and consumption of coagulation factors, platelets, and fibrinolytic proteins secondary to many initiating events, including infection, inflammation, shock, and trauma.

Döhle bodies In Wright-stained peripheral blood films, gray to light blue, round or oval inclusions composed of ribosomal RNA found singly or in multiples near the inner membrane surface of granulocyte cytoplasm.

drepanocyte (sickle cell) Abnormal crescent-shaped red blood cell containing hemoglobin S, characteristic of sickle cell anemia.

drug-induced hemolytic anemia Hemolytic anemia caused directly by a drug or secondary to an antibody-mediated response stimulated by the drug.

dry tap Term used when an inadequate sample of bone marrow fluid is obtained during bone marrow aspiration. Dry taps occur when the marrow is packed, as in chronic myelogenous leukemia, or when it is fibrotic, as in primary myelofibrosis.

dyserythropoiesis Deranged erythropoiesis producing cells with abnormal morphology, as in myelodysplastic syndrome.

dysmegakaryopoiesis Defective megakaryocytic production and maturation characterized by cells with abnormal morphology and increased or decreased megakaryocyte counts.

dysmyelopoiesis Defective myelocytic production and maturation characterized by cells with abnormal morphology; often applied to myelodysplastic syndromes.

dysplasia Abnormal growth pattern; for example, enlarged skull in chronic anemia. Abnormal cervical epithelial cell histopathologic features.

dyspnea Difficult or painful breathing.

echinocyte (burr cell, crenated red blood cell) Red blood cell (RBC) with short, equally spaced, spiny projections. Burr cells are found in uremia and pyruvate kinase deficiency, and observed in all fields of a peripheral blood film. Crenated RBCs are formed by cellular dehydration (drying artifact), and not observed in all fields.

elliptocytes (ovalocytes) Oval red blood cells seen in the peripheral blood in the membrane disorder, hereditary elliptocytosis. May be found in low numbers in healthy states and in other anemias such as iron deficiency and thalassemia.

elliptocytosis (ovalocytosis) Hereditary hematologic disorder characterized by the presence of elliptocytes; often asymptomatic, but may be associated with slight anemia.

Embden–Meyerhof pathway (EMP, glycolysis) A series of enzymatically catalyzed reactions by which glucose and other sugars are metabolized to yield lactic acid (anaerobic glycolysis) or pyruvic acid (aerobic glycolysis). Metabolism releases energy in the form of adenosine triphosphate.

eosinophil Granulocyte with large uniform cytoplasmic granules that stain orange to pink with Wright stain. Granules usually do not obscure the segmented nucleus.

eosinophilia Increase in the blood eosinophil count that is associated with allergies, parasitic infections, or hematologic disorders.

erythrocyte (red blood cell, RBC) Nonnucleated biconcave disk-shaped peripheral blood cell containing hemoglobin. Its primary function is oxygen transport and delivery to tissues.

erythrocytosis Increase in the red blood cell count in peripheral blood.

erythroleukemia Acute malignancy characterized by a proliferation of erythroid and myeloid precursors in bone marrow, and normoblasts with bizarre lobulated nuclei and abnormal myeloblasts in peripheral blood.

erythrophage A phagocyte that has ingested red blood cells.

erythrophagocytosis The ingestion of red blood cells by a macrophage or other phagocyte.

erythropoiesis Bone marrow process of red blood cell production.

erythropoietin (EPO) Glycoprotein hormone synthesized primarily in the kidneys and released into the bloodstream in response to hypoxia. The hormone acts to stimulate and regulate the bone marrow production of red blood cells.

essential thrombocythemia Myeloproliferative neoplasm characterized by marked thrombocytosis and dysfunctional platelets. Patients may experience bleeding or thrombosis.

extramedullary hematopoiesis Production of blood cells outside the bone marrow, such as in the spleen, liver, or lymph nodes. Extramedullary hematopoiesis usually occurs in response to bone marrow fibrosis and loss of bone marrow hematopoiesis.

extravascular hemolysis Destruction of red blood cells outside of a blood vessel, typically by splenic macrophage phagocytosis. Also called macrophage-mediated hemolysis.

faggot cell Promyelocyte containing bundles of Aüer rods sometimes found in acute promyelocytic anemia

flame cell Plasma cell with flame pink cytoplasm owing to presence of IgA

fluorescence in situ hybridization (FISH) Laboratory technique in which fluorescence-labeled nucleic acid probes hybridize to selected DNA or RNA sequences in fixed tissue. FISH allows for the visual microscopic detection of specific polymorphisms or mutations such as BCR/ABL in cell or tissue specimens.

French-American-British (FAB) classification International classification system for acute leukemias, myeloproliferative neoplasms, and myelodysplastic syndromes developed in the 1970s and 1980s. Still in use, although it is being displaced by the World Health Organization classification.

Gaucher disease Rare autosomal recessive disorder of metabolism caused by glucocerebrosidase deficiency and characterized by histiocytic hyperplasia in the liver, spleen, lymph nodes, and bone marrow. The characteristic Gaucher cells, which are lipid-filled macrophages whose cytoplasm resembles crumpled tissue paper, are found on the Wright-stained bone marrow aspirate smear.

glucose–6-phosphate dehydrogenase (G6PD) First enzyme of the glucose monophosphate shunt from the Embden-Meyerhoff pathway. G6PD catalyzes the oxidation of glucose-6-phosphate to a lactone, converting the oxidized form of nicotinamide adenine dinucleotide phosphate (NADP) to the reduced form (NADPH).

glucose–6-phosphate dehydrogenase deficiency X-linked recessive deficiency of glucose-6-phosphate dehydrogenase characterized by episodes of acute intravascular hemolysis under conditions of oxidative stress, including exposure to oxidative drugs such as quinine.

Golgi apparatus Rigid organelle comprised of numerous flattened sacs and associated vesicles. It is the location of the posttranslational modification and storage of glycoproteins, lipoproteins, membrane-bound proteins, and lysosomal enzymes.

gout Painful inflammation caused by excessive plasma uric acid, which becomes deposited as monosodium urate monohydrate in joint capsules and adjacent tendons.

granulocytes Class of white blood cells in peripheral blood characterized by cytoplasmic granules; includes basophils, eosinophils, and neutrophils.

growth factor See cytokines.

hairy cells Malignant B lymphocytes seen in the peripheral blood and bone marrow characterized by delicate gray cytoplasm with projections resembling hairs. These cells are seen in hairy cell leukemia.

Heinz bodies Round blue to purple inclusions attached to inner red blood cell membranes visible when stained with a supravital stain, such as new methylene blue dye. Heinz bodies may be found in multiples, and are composed of precipitated hemoglobin in unstable hemoglobin disorders and glucose-6-phosphate dehydrogenase deficiency.

HELLP syndrome Serious complication of pregnancy with presenting symptoms of hemolysis, elevated liver enzymes, and low platelet count. Peripheral blood morphology is that of microangiopathic hemolytic anemia.

hematoidin Golden yellow, brown, or red crystals that are chemically similar to bilirubin. Hematoidin crystals in a tissue preparation indicate a hemorrhage site.

hematogone Immature B-lymphocyte-like cell appearing in the bone marrow of neonates as a nucleus with indiscernible cytoplasm.

hematology Clinical study of blood cells and blood-forming tissues.

hematopathology Study of the diseases of blood cells and hematopoietic tissue.

hematopoiesis Formation and development of blood cells. Hematopoiesis occurs mostly in the bone marrow and peripheral lymphatic tissues.

hematopoietic stem cell (HSC) Actively dividing cell that is capable of self-renewal and of differentiation into any blood cell lineage.

heme Pigmented iron-containing nonprotein part of the hemoglobin molecule. There are four heme groups in a hemoglobin molecule each containing one ferrous ion in the center. Oxygen binds the ferrous ion and is transported from an area of high to low oxygen concentration.

hemoglobin (Hb, HGB) Tetramer composed of two identical globin chains, each of which binds a heme molecule. Hemoglobin is the primary constituent of red blood cell cytoplasm and transports molecular oxygen from the lungs to the tissues.

hemoglobin C crystal Reddish hexagonal cytoplasmic red blood cell crystal described as a "gold bar," or "Washington monument." Typical of homozygous hemoglobin C disease, crystals form as deoxyhemoglobin C polymerizes.

hemoglobin SC crystal Irregular reddish cytoplasmic red blood cell crystal described as a "glove" or "pistol." Typical of compound heterozygous hemoglobin SC disease, the crystals form as deoxyhemoglobin S and C polymerize.

hemoglobinopathy Condition characterized by structural variations in globin genes that result in the formation of abnormal globin chains. Examples are sickle cell anemia and hemoglobin C disease.

hemolysis Disruption of red blood cell membrane integrity that destroys the cell and releases hemoglobin.

hemolytic anemia Anemia characterized by a shortened red blood cell (RBC) life span and inability of the bone marrow to adequately compensate by increasing RBC synthesis. Hemolytic anemia may be caused by extrinsic or intrinsic disorders.

hemolytic disease of the fetus and newborn (HDFN, erythroblastosis fetalis) Alloimmune anemia caused by maternal IgG antibody that crosses the placenta and binds fetal red blood cell antigens inherited from the father; for instance, maternal anti-A with fetal A antigen. HDFN is characterized by hemolytic anemia, hyperbilirubinemia, and extramedullary erythropoiesis.

hemolytic uremic syndrome (HUS) Severe microangiopathic hemolytic anemia that often follows infection of the gastrointestinal tract by Escherichia coli serotype O157: H7, which produces an exotoxin. It is characterized by renal failure, thrombocytopenia, and the appearance of schistocytes on the peripheral blood film.

hemorrhage Acute severe blood loss often requiring intervention and transfusions.

hemosiderin Intracellular storage form of iron found predominantly in liver, spleen, and bone marrow cells. Hemosiderin is a breakdown product of ferritin that appears in iron overload and hemochromatosis. Hemosiderin may be detected microscopically using the Prussian blue iron stain.

hereditary elliptocytosis (ovalocytosis) Hereditary spectrin defect characterized by the presence of elliptocytes in the peripheral blood; often asymptomatic but may be associated with slight anemia.

hereditary pyropoikilocytosis Rare hereditary defect of spectrin that causes severe hemolytic anemia beginning in childhood, and extreme poikilocytosis with red blood cell morphology resembling that seen in burn patients.

hereditary spherocytosis Hereditary defect in a cytoskeletal or transmembrane protein that results in loss of red blood cell membrane and causes hemolytic anemia characterized by numerous spherocytes on the peripheral blood film.

hereditary stomatocytosis Hereditary defect of the red blood cell membrane resulting in a complex group of diseases in which the hemolysis is mild to severe, and stomatocytes are seen on the peripheral blood film.

heterochromatin The portion of DNA that is inactive during transcription to messenger RNA and stains deeply with Wright stain.

heterozygous Having two different alleles at corresponding loci on homologous chromosomes. An individual who is heterozygous for a trait has inherited an allele for that trait from one parent and an alternative allele from the other parent. A person who is heterozygous for a genetic disease will manifest the disorder if it is caused by a dominant allele, but will remain asymptomatic if the disease is caused by a recessive allele.

histiocyte (macrophage) Mononuclear phagocyte found in all tissues; part of the immune system.

homozygous Having two identical alleles at corresponding loci on homologous chromosomes. An individual who is homozygous for a trait has inherited one identical allele for that trait from each parent. A person who is homozygous for a genetic disease caused by a pair of recessive alleles manifests the disorder.

Howell-Jolly (H-J) bodies Round blue to purple inclusions in red blood cells (RBCs), usually one per RBC, visible on Wright-stained peripheral blood films. Howell-Jolly bodies are composed of DNA and may indicate severe anemia or splenectomy.

hypercellular bone marrow Bone marrow showing an abnormal increase in the concentration of nucleated hematopoietic cells; potentially associated with leukemia or hemolytic anemia.

hypersegmented neutrophil Neutrophil with six or more nuclear lobes or segments; often associated with megaloblastic anemia.

hypersplenism Increased hemolytic activity of the spleen caused by splenomegaly resulting in deficiency of peripheral blood cells and compensatory hypercellularity of the bone marrow.

hypocellular bone marrow Abnormal decrease in the number of nucleated hematopoietic cells present in the bone marrow; may be associated with aplastic anemia or fibrosis.

hypochromia Abnormal decrease in the hemoglobin content of red blood cells so that they appear pale, with a larger central pallor when stained with Wright stain. These cells are called hypochromic.

immune hemolytic anemia Anemia resulting from shortened red blood cell (RBC) life span caused by antibodies to RBC membrane antigens or complement. The immunoglobulin or complement-coated RBCs are cleared by splenic macrophages. Anemia results when the bone marrow fails to compensate for RBC consumption.

immunoglobulin (antibody) Protein of the γ-globulin fraction produced by B lymphocytes and plasma cells that recognizes and binds a specific antigen. Immunoglobulins are the basis of humoral immunity.

immunophenotyping Classification of white blood cells and platelets by their membrane antigens. Synthetic antibodies, often monoclonal antibodies produced by hybridoma technology, are used to identify the antigens in flow cytometry.

infectious mononucleosis Acute infection caused by the Epstein-Barr virus, a herpesvirus. Characterized by fever, sore throat, lymphadenopathy, variant lymphocytes, splenomegaly, hepatomegaly, abnormal liver function, and bruising. Laboratory tests used to identify the disease include blood film review for reactive lymphocytes, serologic mononucleosis testing, and molecular identification of the Epstein-Barr virus.

intracranial hemorrhage (ICH, hemorrhagic stroke) Bleeding into the brain causing tissue death.

intramedullary hematopoiesis Formation and development of blood cells within the marrow cavity of a bone.

intravascular hemolysis Red blood cell destruction that occurs within the blood vessels at a rate exceeding splenic macrophage clearance capacity, releasing hemoglobin into the plasma. Seen in acute hemolytic episodes such as those associated with transfusion reaction, glucose-6-phosphate dehydrogenase deficiency, and sickle cell anemia crisis.

iron deficiency anemia Microcytic, hypochromic anemia caused by inadequate supplies of the iron needed to synthesize hemoglobin and characterized by pallor, fatigue, and weakness. Often caused by low dietary iron intake or chronic blood loss.

leukemia Group of malignant neoplasms of hematopoietic tissues characterized by diffuse replacement of bone marrow or lymph nodes, with abnormal proliferating white blood cells and the presence of leukemic cells in the peripheral blood. Leukemia may be chronic or acute, and myeloid or lymphoid.

leukemoid reaction Clinical syndrome resembling leukemia in which the white blood cell count is elevated to greater than $50,000/\mu l$ in response to an allergen, inflammatory disease, infection, poison, hemorrhage, burn, or severe physical stress. Leukemoid reaction usually involves granulocytes and is distinguished from chronic myelogenous leukemia by the use of the leukocyte alkaline phosphatase staining of neutrophils.

leukocyte One of the formed elements of the blood. The five families of WBCs are lymphocytes, monocytes, neutrophils, basophils, and eosinophils. WBCs function as: phagocytes of bacteria, fungi, and viruses; detoxifiers of toxic proteins that may be produced by allergic reactions and cellular injury; and immune system cells.

leukocytosis Abnormally elevated white blood cell count in peripheral blood.

lymphoblast Immature cell found in the bone marrow and lymph nodes, but not normally in the peripheral blood; the most primitive, morphologically recognizable precursor in the lymphocytic series, which develops into the prolymphocyte.

lymphocytes Mononuclear, nonphagocytic white blood cells found in the blood, lymph, and lymphoid tissues. Lymphocytes are categorized as B and T lymphocytes and natural killer cells. They are responsible for humoral and cellular immunity, and tumor surveillance.

lymphocytopenia (lymphopenia) Abnormally reduced lymphocyte count in peripheral blood.

lymphocytosis Abnormally increased lymphocyte count in peripheral blood.

lymphoid Resembling or pertaining to lymph, or tissue and cells of the lymphoid system.

lymphoma Solid tumor neoplasm of lymphoid tissue categorized as Hodgkin or non-Hodgkin lymphoma, and defined by lymphocyte morphology and the histologic features of the lymph nodes.

lymphoproliferative Pertaining to the proliferation of lymphoid cells resulting in abnormally increased lymphocyte counts in peripheral blood indicating a reactive or neoplastic condition.

lysosomes Membrane-bound sacs of varying size distributed randomly in the cytoplasm of granulocytes and platelets. Lysosomes contain hydrolytic enzymes that kill ingested bacteria, and digest bacteria and other foreign materials.

macrocyte Red blood cell with an abnormally large diameter seen on a peripheral blood film, and an elevated mean cell volume. Associated with folate and vitamin B12 deficiency, bone marrow failure, myelodysplastic syndrome, and chronic liver disease.

macroglobulin High-molecular-weight plasma globulin, such as α-2-macroglobulin or an immunoglobulin of the M isotype. Abnormal monoclonal IgM proteins seen in Waldenström macroglobulinemia.

macrophage (histiocyte) Mononuclear phagocyte found in all tissues; part of the immune system.

malaria Infectious disease caused by one or more of five species of the protozoan genus Plasmodium. Malaria is transmitted from human to human by a bite from an infected Anopheles mosquito.

malignant Describes a cancerous disease that threatens life through its ability to metastasize.

mast cell Connective tissue cell that has large basophilic granules containing heparin, serotonin, bradykinin, and histamine. These substances are released from the mast cell in response to immunoglobulin E stimulation.

May–Hegglin anomaly Rare autosomal dominant disorder characterized by thrombocytopenia and granulocytes that contain cytoplasmic inclusions similar to Döhle bodies.

mean cell hemoglobin (MCH) Average red blood cell (RBC) hemoglobin mass in picograms computed from the RBC count and hemoglobin level.

mean cell hemoglobin concentration (MCHC) Average relative hemoglobin concentration per red blood cell (RBC), expressed in g/dl, and computed from the hemoglobin and hematocrit. Relates to Wright-stained RBC color intensity.

mean cell volume (MCV) Average red blood cell (RBC) volume in femtoliters computed from the RBC count and hematocrit, or directly measured by an automated hematology analyzer. Relates to Wright-stained RBC diameter.

megakaryoblast Least differentiated visually identifiable megakaryocyte precursor in a Wright-stained bone marrow aspirate smear. The megakaryoblast cannot be distinguished visually from the myeloblast, but is identified using special immunochemical markers.

megakaryocyte Largest cell in the bone marrow measuring 30 to 50 μm and having a multilobed nucleus. Its cytoplasm is composed of platelets, which are released to the blood through the extension of proplatelet processes. Megakaryocytes are identified and enumerated microscopically at low (10×) power on a bone marrow aspirate smear.

megaloblast Abnormally large, nucleated, immature precursor of the erythrocytic series; an abnormal counterpart to the pronormoblast. Not only does it have a larger diameter, but the nucleus appears more immature than the cytoplasm. Megaloblasts give rise to macrocytic red blood cells and are associated with megaloblastic anemia, usually caused by folate or vitamin B_{12} deficiency.

metamyelocyte Stage in the development of the granulocyte series located between the myelocyte stage and the band stage. Characterized by mature, granulated cytoplasm, and a bean-shaped nucleus.

metarubricyte (orthochromatic normoblast) Fourth stage of bone marrow erythropoiesis and the last in which the cell retains a nucleus. The nucleus is fully condensed with no parachromatin, and the cytoplasm is 85% hemoglobinized, and bluish-pink. When an orthochromatic normoblast appears in the peripheral blood, it is called a nucleated red blood cell.

metastasis Extension or spread of tumor cells to distant parts of the body, usually through the lymphatics or blood vessels.

microangiopathic hemolytic anemia (MAHA) Condition in which narrowing or obstruction of small blood vessels by fibrin or platelet aggregates results in distortion and fragmentation of red blood cells, hemolysis, and anemia. This causes the appearance of schistocytes on a Wright-stained blood film.

microcyte Small red blood cell (RBC) with reduced mean cell volume and reduced diameter on Wright-stained peripheral blood film. Microcytes are often associated with iron deficiency anemia and thalassemia.

mitochondria Round or oval structures distributed randomly in the cytoplasm of a cell. Mitochondria provide the cell's aerobic energy system by producing adenosine triphosphate.

mitosis Ordinary process of somatic cell division resulting in the production of two daughter cells that have identical diploid complements of chromosomes.

monoblast The most undifferentiated morphologically identifiable precursor of the bone marrow monocytic series; develops into the promonocyte.

monoclonal Pertaining to or designating a group of identical cells or organisms derived from a single cell or organism. Also used to describe products from a clone of cells such as monoclonal antibodies.

monocyte Mononuclear phagocytic white blood cell having a round to horseshoe-shaped nucleus, with abundant gray-blue cytoplasm, and filled with fine reddish granules. Circulating precursor to the macrophage, the primary phagocytic cell of most tissues.

mononuclear Having only one nucleus. Used to describe cells such as monocytes or lymphocytes as distinct from neutrophils, which have nuclei that appear to be multiple and hence are called segmented or polymorphonuclear.

Mott cell Plasma cell containing colorless cytoplasmic inclusions of immunoglobulin called Russell bodies that appear similar to vacuoles.

multiple myeloma (now called plasma cell myeloma) Malignant neoplasm in which plasma cells proliferate in the bone marrow, destroying bone and resulting in pain, fractures, and excess production of a monoclonal plasma immunoglobulin.

myelo- Prefix relating to the bone marrow or spinal cord and used to identify granulocytic precursors of neutrophils.

myeloblast Least differentiated morphologically identifiable bone marrow precursor of the granulocytic series; develops into the promyelocyte. The appearance of myeloblasts in peripheral blood signals acute leukemia.

myelocyte Third stage of bone marrow granulocytic series differentiation, intermediate in development between a promyelocyte and a metamyelocyte. In this stage, differentiation of cytoplasmic granules has begun, so myelocytes may be basophilic, eosinophilic, or neutrophilic.

myelodysplastic syndromes (MDSs) Group of acquired clonal hematologic disorders characterized by progressive peripheral blood cytopenias that reflect defects in erythroid, myeloid, or megakaryocytic maturation.

myelofibrosis Replacement of bone marrow with fibrous connective tissue.

myeloid General term used to denote granulocytic cells and their precursors including basophils, eosinophils, and neutrophils. Lymphoid and erythroid cell lines are excluded, and most morphologists also exclude the monocytic and megakaryocytic cell lines.

myeloid-to-erythroid (M:E) ratio Proportion of myeloid cells to nucleated erythroid precursors in bone marrow aspirate. The myeloid-to-erythroid ratio is used to evaluate hematologic cell production. Excluded from the myeloid cell count are monocytic and lymphoid precursors and plasma cells.

myeloperoxidase (MPO) Enzyme that occurs in primary granules of promyelocytes, myelocytes, and neutrophils and exhibits bactericidal, fungicidal, and virucidal properties.

Cytochemical stains that detect myeloperoxidase are used to identify myeloid precursors in acute leukemia.

myeloproliferative neoplasms (MPN, myeloproliferative disorders, MPD) Group of neoplasms characterized by proliferation of myeloid tissue and elevations in one or more myeloid cell types in the peripheral blood. Myeloproliferative neoplasms include primary myelofibrosis, essential thrombocythemia, polycythemia vera, and chronic myelogenous leukemia.

necrosis Localized tissue death that occurs in groups of cells in response to disease or injury.

neonatal Pertaining to the first 28 days after birth.

neoplasm Any abnormal growth of new tissue; can be malignant or benign. The term is usually applied to cancerous cells.

neutrophil Mature segmented (polymorphonuclear) white blood cell with fine pink-staining cytoplasmic granules in a Wright-stained peripheral blood film. Neutrophils ingest bacteria and cellular debris.

normochromic Describes a Wright-stained red blood cell with normal color and normal hemoglobin content and a mean cell hemoglobin concentration within the reference interval.

normocyte Normal, mature red blood cell with a mean cell volume within the reference interval.

nucleated red blood cell (NRBC) Red blood cell (RBC) in peripheral blood that possesses a nucleus; often an orthochromic normoblast (metarubricyte).

nucleolus Round or irregular pocket of messenger and ribosomal RNA in the nucleus. Nucleoli are observed by morphologists and are used to distinguish cell differentiation stages.

nucleus Cellular organelle containing DNA and RNA. Stores genetic information and controls cell functions.

nucleus-to-cytoplasm (N:C) ratio Estimated volume of a Wright-stained nucleus in comparison to the volume of the cytoplasm. The nucleus-to-cytoplasm ratio is used to differentiate cell developmental stages.

objective Microscope lens closest to the specimen. Most clinical grade microscopes provide $10 \times$ dry, $40 \times$ dry or $50 \times$ oil immersion, and $100 \times$ oil immersion objectives.

orthochromic normoblast (metarubricyte) Fourth stage of bone marrow erythropoiesis and the last in which the cell retains a nucleus. The nucleus is fully condensed with no parachromatin; the cytoplasm is 85% hemoglobinized and bluish-pink. When an orthochromic normoblast appears in the peripheral blood, it is called a nucleated red blood cell.

osteoblast Bone-forming cell.

osteoclast Large multinuclear cell associated with the absorption and removal of bone. May be confused with a megakaryocyte.

oval macrocyte Oval red blood cell with an increased diameter seen in peripheral blood. Characteristic of megaloblastic anemia.

ovalocyte (elliptocyte) Oval red blood cell seen in peripheral blood in the membrane disorder hereditary elliptocytosis. May be found in low numbers in healthy states and in other anemias such as iron deficiency and thalassemia major.

pancytopenia Marked reduction in the count of red blood cells, white blood cells, and platelets in peripheral blood.

Pappenheimer bodies (siderotic granules) Red blood cell inclusions composed of ferric iron. On Prussian blue iron stain preparations they appear as multiple dark blue irregular granules. On Wright stain preparations they appear as pale blue clusters.

parachromatin Pale-staining portion of the nucleus, roughly equivalent to euchromatin.

Pelger-Huët anomaly Autosomal dominant, asymptomatic anomaly of neutrophil nuclei, which fail to segment and appear dumbbell shaped or peanut shaped ("pince-nez" nuclei). Pelgeroid nuclei are more common and resemble the nuclei of Pelger-Huët anomaly, but may indicate myelodysplasia, or may appear during chemotherapy.

perinuclear hof or halo A clear area occurring near the nucleus of a cell such as a plasma cell.

pernicious anemia Progressive autoimmune disorder that results in megaloblastic macrocytic anemia because of a lack of, or antibodies to, parietal cells or intrinsic factor essential for the absorption of vitamin B12.

phagocyte Cell that is able to surround, engulf, and digest microorganisms and cellular debris. Macrophages and neutrophils are phagocytes.

phagocytosis Ingestion of large particles or live microorganisms into a cell.

Philadelphia chromosome Reciprocal translocation of the long arm of chromosome 22 to chromosome 9; definitive for the diagnosis of chronic myelogenous leukemia. The mutation results in the fusion of the BCR and ABL genes, and abnormal tyrosine kinase production.

phlebotomy Use of a needle to puncture a vein and collect blood.

plasma cell Fully differentiated B lymphocyte found in the bone marrow and lymphoid tissue, and occasionally in peripheral blood. It contains an eccentric nucleus with deeply staining chromatin and abundant dark blue cytoplasm. The Golgi apparatus produces a perinuclear halo resulting from its high lipid content. Plasma cells secrete antibodies in the humoral immune response.

platelet (thrombocyte) Smallest of the formed elements in blood; disk-shaped, 2 to 4 μm in diameter, nonnucleated cell formed in the bone marrow from the cytoplasm of megakaryocytes. Platelets trigger and control blood coagulation.

platelet satellitism (satellitosis) Antibody-mediated in vitro adhesion of platelets to segmented neutrophils. Occurs primarily in specimens anticoagulated with ethylenediaminetetraacetic acid (EDTA) and causes pseudothrombocytopenia.

pleomorphic Occurring in various distinct forms; having the ability to exist in various forms and to change from one form to another.

pluripotential stem cell Stem cell that has the potential to differentiate into one of several types of hematopoietic progenitor cells, including lymphocytic, monocytic, granulocytic, megakaryocytic, and erythrocytic lineages, in addition to nonhematopoietic cells.

poikilocytosis Presence of red blood cells with varying or bizarre shapes in the peripheral blood.

polychromatic (polychromatophilic) Having a staining quality in which both acid and basic stains are incorporated. Usually used to denote a mixture of pink and blue in the cytoplasm of Wright-stained cells.

polychromatic normoblast (polychromatophilic normoblast, rubricyte) Precursor in the erythrocytic maturation series, intermediate between the basophilic normoblast (prorubricyte) and the orthochromic normoblast (metarubricyte). In this stage, differentiation is based on the decreasing cell diameter and the gray-blue cytoplasm as hemoglobin first becomes visible by Wright stain.

polychromatic or polychromatophilic red blood cell (reticulocyte) Immature but anucleate red blood cell (RBC) with bluish-pink cytoplasm on a Wright-stained blood film. When new methylene blue dye is used, the cytoplasm of these cells has a meshlike pattern of dark blue threads and particles, vestiges of the endoplasmic reticulum. Reticulocytosis or polychromatophilia indicates bone marrow regeneration activity in hemolytic anemia or acute blood loss.

polychromatophilia (reticulocytosis) Elevated reticulocyte count on a peripheral blood film stained with new methylene blue dye, or an increase in the number of polychromatophilic red blood cells on a Wright-stained blood film. Reticulocytosis or polychromatophilia indicates bone marrow regeneration activity in hemolytic anemia or acute blood loss.

polycythemia (erythrocytosis) Elevated red blood cell count, hemoglobin, and hematocrit in peripheral blood, usually in response to chronic hypoxia.

polycythemia vera (PV) Myeloproliferative neoplasm in which a somatic mutation leads to a marked increase in the red blood cell (RBC) count, hematocrit, hemoglobin, white blood cell count, platelet count, and red blood cell mass. RBC precursors are hypersensitive to erythropoietin.

polymorphonuclear neutrophil (PMN, segmented neutrophil, seg) White blood cell whose nucleus is condensed into two to five segments or lobes connected by filaments. Distinguished from mononuclear cells such as monocytes and lymphocytes.

precursor Differentiating (immature) hematopoietic cell stage that is morphologically identifiable as belonging to a given cell line; for example, pronormoblasts (rubriblasts) are precursors of basophilic normoblasts (prorubricytes) in erythropoiesis.

progenitor Undifferentiated (immature) hematopoietic cell that is committed to a cell line, but cannot be identified morphologically.

prolymphocyte Developmental form in the lymphocytic series that is intermediate between the lymphoblast and the lymphocyte.

promegakaryocyte Morphologically identifiable bone marrow cell stage that is intermediate between the megakaryoblast and the megakaryocyte.

promonocyte Precursor in the monocytic series; the cell stage intermediate in development between the monoblast and the monocyte.

promyelocyte Precursor in the granulocytic (myelocytic) series that is intermediate in development between a myeloblast and a myelocyte; contains primary granules.

pronormoblast (rubriblast) Undifferentiated (immature) hematopoietic cell that is the most primitive morphologically identifiable precursor in the erythrocytic series; differentiates into the basophilic normoblast (prorubricyte).

prorubricyte (basophilic normoblast) Second identifiable stage in bone marrow erythrocytic maturation; it is derived from the pronormoblast (rubriblast). Typically 10 to 15 μm in diameter, the prorubricyte has cytoplasm that stains dark blue with Wright stain.

Pseudo-Gaucher-cells They resemble Gaucher cells and are found in the bone marrow of some patients with thalassemia major, chronic myelogenous leukemia, and acute lymphoblastic leukemia. However, the cells result from the glucocerebrosidase enzyme being overwhelmed by rapid cell turnover, rather than a decrease in glucocerebrosidase.

pseudo-gout A condition causing symptoms similar to gout, but caused by calcium pyrophosphate crystals in joints as opposed to the monosodium urate crystals of gout.

pseudo–Pelger-Huët cell (Pelgeroid cell) Hyposegmented, hypogranular neutrophils that resemble Pelger-Huët cells. Helpful in the diagnosis of leukemia, myeloproliferative neoplasms, and myelodysplastic syndromes.

pyknosis Degeneration of a cell in which the nucleus shrinks in size and the chromatin condenses to a solid, structureless mass or masses. It is part of the process of apoptosis, or is indicative of the effects of chemotherapy.

pyropoikilocytosis (hereditary pyropoikilocytosis) Rare hereditary defect of spectrin that causes severe hemolytic anemia beginning in childhood, with extreme poikilocytosis in which the red blood cell morphology resembles that seen in burn patients.

pyruvate kinase (PK) Enzyme that converts phosphoenolpyruvate to pyruvate generating two molecules of ATP; essential for aerobic and anaerobic glycolysis.

pyruvate kinase deficiency Autosomal recessive disorder resulting in a deficiency of pyruvate kinase, the enzyme that converts phosphoenolpyruvate to pyruvate; causes hemolytic anemia by reducing red blood cell life span. It is the most common enzyme deficiency of the Embden-Meyerhof pathway.

reactive lymphocytes (variant, transformed, or atypical lymphocytes) Lymphocytes whose altered morphology includes stormy blue cytoplasm, and lobular or irregular nuclei. Variant lymphocytes indicate stimulation by a virus, particularly Epstein-Barr virus, which causes infectious mononucleosis.

red blood cell (RBC) indices Numerical representations of average RBC volume (mean cell volume), hemoglobin mass (mean cell hemoglobin), and relative hemoglobin concentration (mean cell hemoglobin concentration). Indices are computed from the RBC count, hemoglobin, and hematocrit values. The mean cell volume is directly measured by some hematology analyzers.

red cell distribution width (RDW) Coefficient of variation of red blood cell volume as measured by an electronic cell counter. An increased red cell distribution width indicates anisocytosis.

red marrow Hematopoietic bone marrow, in contrast to yellow, fatty bone marrow.

reticulocyte (polychromatic or polychromatophilic red blood cell) Immature but anuclate red blood cell (RBC) that shows a meshlike pattern of dark blue threads and particles, vestiges of the endoplasmic reticulum, when stained with new methylene blue vital dye. In a Wright-stained blood film, no filaments are seen but the cytoplasm stains bluish-pink and the cell is called a polychromatic or polychromatophilic RBC. Reticulocytosis or polychromatophilia indicates bone marrow regeneration activity in hemolytic anemia or acute blood loss.

reticulocytosis (polychromatophilia) Elevated reticulocyte count on a peripheral blood film stained with new methylene blue dye or increase in the number of polychromatophilic red blood cells on a Wright-stained blood film. Reticulocytosis or polychromatophilia indicates bone marrow regeneration activity in hemolytic anemia or acute blood loss.

Rhnull disease Hemolytic anemia in persons who lack all Rh antigens (Rhnull); marked by spherocytosis, stomatocytosis, and increased osmotic fragility.

ribonucleic acid (RNA) Single strand of polynucleotides connected by ribose molecules. RNA base sequences are transcribed from DNA, and are the basis for translation to proteins. Major types of RNA include messenger RNA, ribosomal RNA, and transfer RNA.

ribosomes Granules embedded in the membranes of endoplasmic reticulum that are composed of protein and RNA. Ribosomes are the sites for primary protein translation from messenger and transfer RNA.

ring sideroblast Nucleated red blood cell precursor with at least five iron granules that circle at least one third of the nucleus. These cells, visible with Prussian blue stain, are the pathognomonic finding in refractory anemia with ring sideroblasts.

Romanowsky stain Prototype of the many eosin–methylene blue stains for blood cells and malarial parasites, including Wright and Giemsa stain.

rouleaux Aggregation of stacked red blood cells caused by elevated plasma proteins and abnormal monoclonal proteins.

rubriblast (pronormoblast) Undifferentiated (immature) hematopoietic cell that is the most primitive morphologically identifiable precursor in the erythrocytic series; differentiates into the basophilic normoblast (prorubricyte).

rubricyte (polychromatic or polychromatophilic normoblast) Precursor in the erythrocytic maturation series that is intermediate between the basophilic normoblast (prorubricyte) and the orthochromic normoblast (metarubricyte). In this stage, differentiation is based on the decreasing cell diameter and the gray-blue cytoplasm as hemoglobin first becomes visible.

schistocyte (schizocyte) Fragmented red blood cell characteristic of microangiopathic hemolytic anemia, severe burns, disseminated intravascular coagulation, and prosthetic mechanical trauma.

segmented neutrophil (seg, polymorphonuclear neutrophil, PMN) White blood cell whose nucleus is condensed into two to five segments connected by filaments. Distinguished from mononuclear cells such as monocytes and lymphocytes.

Sézary cell Mononuclear cell with a cerebriform nucleus (resembling the surface of the cerebrum) and a narrow rim of cytoplasm. It is a characteristic finding in cutaneous T-cell lymphomas.

Sézary syndrome Cutaneous T-cell lymphoma characterized by exfoliative erythroderma, peripheral lymphadenopathy, and the presence of Sézary cells in the skin, lymph nodes, and peripheral blood.

sickle cell (drepanocyte) Abnormal crescent-shaped red blood cell containing hemoglobin S, characteristic of sickle cell anemia.

sickle cell anemia (sickle cell disease) Severe chronic hemoglobinopathy in people who are homozygous for hemoglobin S. The abnormal hemoglobin results in distortion of red blood cells (sickle cells) and leads to crises characterized by joint pain, anemia, thrombosis, fever, and splenomegaly.

sickle cell crisis Any of several acute conditions occurring as part of sickle cell disease as follows: aplastic crisis, which is temporary bone marrow aplasia; hemolytic crisis, which is acute red blood cell destruction; and vasoocclusive crisis, which is severe pain due to blockage of the blood vessels.

sickle cell trait Asymptomatic heterozygous condition characterized by the presence of both hemoglobin S and hemoglobin A.

sideroblast Bone marrow erythrocytic precursor that shows excessive iron granules (siderotic granules) with Prussian blue staining.

siderocyte Nonnucleated red blood cell in which particles of iron (siderotic granules) are visible with Prussian blue staining.

siderotic granules (Pappenheimer bodies) Red blood cell inclusions composed of ferric iron. With Prussian blue iron staining, they appear as multiple dark blue irregular granules.

spectrin Major cytoskeletal protein forming a lattice at the cytoplasmic surface of the cell membrane, providing lateral support to the membrane and thus maintaining its shape. Abnormalities in red blood cell spectrin account for hereditary spherocytosis, ovalocytosis, and pyropoikilocytosis.

spherocyte Abnormal spherical red blood cell with a decreased surface area-to-volume ratio. In Wright-stained peripheral blood films, spherocytes are dense, lack central pallor, and have a reduced diameter. Spherocytes appear most frequently in warm autoimmune hemolytic anemia and hereditary spherocytosis.

spleen Large organ in the upper left quadrant of the abdomen, just under the stomach. The spleen has the body's largest collection of macrophages, which are responsible for phagocytosis and elimination of senescent red blood cells. The spleen also houses many lymphoid cells.

splenectomy Excision of the spleen.

stem cell Undifferentiated mononuclear cell whose daughter cells may give rise to a variety of cell types and which is capable of renewing itself and thus maintaining a pool of cells that can differentiate into multiple other cell types.

stomatocyte Abnormal cup-shaped mature red blood cell that has a slitlike area of central pallor.

supravital stain (vital stain) Stain that colors living tissues or cells.

systemic lupus erythematosus (SLE) Chronic autoimmune inflammatory disease manifested by severe vasculitis, renal involvement, and lesions of the skin and nervous system.

T cell (T lymphocyte) Lymphocyte that participates in cellular immunity, including cell-to-cell communication. The major T cell categories are helper cells and suppressor-cytotoxic cells.

target cell (codocyte) Poorly hemoglobinized red blood cell (RBC) that is present in hemoglobinopathies, thalassemia, and liver disease. In a Wright-stained peripheral blood film, hemoglobin concentrates in the center of the RBC and around the periphery to resemble a "bull's-eye."

teardrop cell (dacryocyte) Red blood cell with a single pointed extension, resembling a teardrop. Dacryocytes are often seen in the myeloproliferative neoplasm called myelofibrosis with myeloid metaplasia.

thalassemia Production and hemolytic anemia characterized by microcytic, hypochromic red

thrombocyte Platelet.

thrombocythemia Abnormally high platelet count with dysfunctional platelets; seen in the myeloproliferative neoplasm known as essential thrombocythemia.

thrombocytopenia Platelet count below the lower limit of the reference interval, usually 150,000/μl.

thrombocytosis Platelet count above the upper limit of the reference interval, usually 450,000/μl.

thrombotic thrombocytopenic purpura (TTP) Congenital or acquired deficiency of ADAMTS-13, an endothelial cell— von Willebrand factor-cleaving protease. Ultra-large von Willebrand factor multimers activate platelets to form white clots in the microvasculature, causing severe thrombocytopenia, with mucocutaneous bleeding, microangiopathic hemolytic anemia, and neuropathy.

toxic granulation Presence of abnormally large, dark-staining, or dominant primary granules in neutrophils associated with bacterial infections.

vacuole Any clear space or cavity formed in the cytoplasm of a cell.

vacuolization Formation of vacuoles.

venipuncture Use of a needle to puncture a vein and collect blood.

vital stain (supravital stain) Stain that colors living tissues or cells.

vitamin B_{12} (cyanocobalamin) Complex vitamin involved in the metabolism of protein, fats, and carbohydrate; normal blood formation; and nerve function.

Waldenström macroglobulinemia Form of monoclonal gammopathy in which IgM is overproduced by the clone of a plasma cell. Increased viscosity of the blood may result in circulatory impairment, and normal immunoglobulin synthesis is decreased, which increases susceptibility to infections.

warm antibody IgG antibody that reacts optimally at a temperature of 37° C.

warm autoimmune hemolytic anemia Most common autoimmune hemolytic anemia, which results from the reaction of IgG autoantibodies with red blood cells at an optimal temperature of 37° C.

COMPARISON TABLES

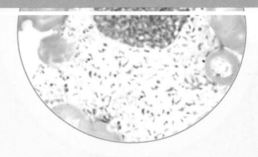

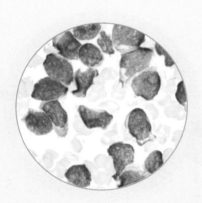

TABLE A-1

Lymphocyte versus Neutrophilic Myelocyte

	Lymphocyte	Myelocyte
Shape	Round to oval	Usually oval
Size	10-18 μm	12-18 μm
Nucleus	Round to oval; may be slightly indented	Round to oval; slightly eccentric; may have one flattened side; may be a clearing next to the nucleus in the Golgi area
Nucleoli	Occasional	Usually not visible
Chromatin	Condensed; clumpy; blocky; smudged	Coarse and slightly condensed
Cytoplasm	Scant to moderate; sky blue; may be more blue at edges	Slightly basophilic to lavender/pink
Granules	May be a few azurophilic	Primary: few to moderate Secondary: variable number; become more predominant as cell matures
Vacuoles	Occasional	None
Examples		

TABLE A-2

Monocyte versus Reactive Lymphocyte

	Monocyte	Reactive Lymphocyte
Shape	Pleomorphic; may have pseudopodia, which tend to "push away" surrounding cells	Pleomorphic, easily indented by surrounding cells
Size	12-20 μm	10-30 μm
Nucleus	Round, oval, horseshoe, or kidney shaped, may have brainlike convolutions	Irregular, elongated, stretched, occasionally round
Nucleoli	Absent	Occasionally present
Chromatin	Loosely woven, lacy	Variable; coarse to fine and dispersed
Cytoplasm	Blue-gray	Pale blue to deeply basophilic, may stain unevenly
Granules	Many fine red—may give ground glass appearance	May be a few prominent azurophilic granules
Vacuoles	Absent to numerous	Occasional
Examples		

Use as many criteria as possible to identify cells. It is often difficult to differentiate cells in isolation; multiple fields should be examined for nuclear and cytoplasmic characteristics. Consider "the company they keep."

INDEX

Note: Page numbers followed by *f* indicate figures, *b* indicate boxes and *t* indicate tables.